Praise for *Trusting the Dawn*

"*Trusting the Dawn* bridges the story of a real-life trauma with the practical tools to transform yourself and your life. This book is medicine for anyone who wants to free their mind, body, and soul from the past."

DR. JOE DISPENZA

New York Times bestselling author of *You Are the Placebo* and *Becoming Supernatural*

"Mary's vulnerability in sharing her healing journey from trauma to thriving is an absolute inspiration. In *Trusting the Dawn*, she provides valuable resources for anyone touched by trauma to effectively heal and transform."

KELLY NOONAN GORES

author and producer/director of the acclaimed *Heal* documentary

"For anyone who has experienced trauma on any level, Mary Firestone's words will serve as a beacon of hope—a road map to finding your way back to a new normal and living life to its fullest. This book will stay on your bedside table for years after you read the last word."

LYDIA FENET

bestselling author of *The Most Powerful Woman in the Room Is You*

"I am blown away by Mary's bravery in sharing her vulnerability in order to heal after trauma. Her journey will undoubtedly help others to recognize that they are not alone, that there are many ways out and through to the other side. Her candor and heartfelt, sage wisdom reframe trauma as an asset you can reappropriate as strength to lead a better life."

JILL KARGMAN

author, writer, and actress

"Mary's brilliant reframing of trauma in *Trusting the Dawn* is an inspiration to us all to live a more authentic and joyful life. Mary embodies what it means to emerge transformed, owning the phrase 'What if this is happening for us, not to us?' Mary's book debut is a must-read, a road map through trauma to transformation, and an essential tool kit for our lives."

LAUREN ROXBURGH

bestselling author and presenter

"Mary Firestone is a leader of growth consciousness. She has a heart as big as the moon and is equally as brilliant. What makes Mary a true influence in my life is her willingness to do the work, work the love, and transform pain into purpose. She is a shining star of talent and grit."

DR. JENNIFER FREED

author and celebrity psychological astrologer

"Through our willingness to breathe in the dark, we are able to find the light. Mary shows others that finding their light in the darkness is possible. And it's even brighter than before it went dark."

SHAMAN DUREK

author of *Spirit Hacking* and *Alchemy Elementals*

TRUSTING
THE
DAWN

TRUSTING THE DAWN

How to Choose Freedom and Joy After Trauma

MARY FIRESTONE

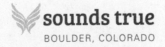

sounds true

BOULDER, COLORADO

Sounds True
Boulder, CO 80306

This book is not intended as a substitute for the medical recommendations of physicians,
mental health professionals, or other health-care providers. Rather, it is intended to offer
information to help the reader cooperate with physicians, mental health professionals,
and health-care providers in a mutual quest for optimal well-being. We advise readers to
carefully review and understand the ideas presented and to seek the advice of a qualified
professional before attempting to use them.

Published 2022

Book design by Linsey Dodaro

Printed in the United States of America

BK06382

Library of Congress Cataloging-in-Publication Data
Names: Firestone, Mary, 1977- author.
Title: Trusting the dawn : how to choose freedom and joy after trauma /
    Mary Firestone.
Description: Boulder, CO : Sounds True, [2022] | Includes bibliographical
    references.
Identifiers: LCCN 2021053330 (print) | LCCN 2021053331 (ebook) | ISBN
    9781683649120 (hardcover) | ISBN 9781683649137 (ebook)
Subjects: LCSH: Firestone, Mary, 1977- | Psychic trauma--Alternative
    treatment. | Traumatic incident reduction. | Psychotherapy. | Mind and
    body.
Classification: LCC RC552.T7 F556 2022 (print) | LCC RC552.T7 (ebook) |
    DDC 616.85/21--dc23/eng/20220309
LC record available at https://lccn.loc.gov/2021053330
LC ebook record available at https://lccn.loc.gov/2021053331

10 9 8 7 6 5 4 3 2 1

To all who are struggling in the dark aftermath of trauma:

Dawn is breaking.

It is dark before the dawn,
but the dawn never fails.
Trust in the dawn.

FLORENCE SCOVEL SHINN

Contents

Introduction

It was more than five hours before I was rescued from my bathroom countertop, where I huddled, wet and pregnant, shaking from cold and fear, trapped by millions of gallons of mud. I didn't know how many hours I'd endure in this soggy, frigid tomb; I did know they seemed both interminable and fleeting. For much of that time, I thought my husband and four-year-old son had been swept away in a river of mud and debris and that my own death was imminent.

In mere moments, the tidal wave of mud had become too high and toxic for me to stand in, so I had crawled up on the countertop. Barefoot, in thin cotton floral pajamas, I looked out my bathroom window at my world, destroyed. I thought my life was over. There had been a deafening roar as boulders the size of tanks tumbled in a torrential river of mud down the mountain above my home. On my left, I had watched this river crumple a neighbor's house and hurtle it down the hill away from me. On my right, the majority of my house had twisted backward and washed away at twenty miles per hour. Not only was my living room gone but my panic surpassed anything I'd ever known when I realized the window looking back at me was that of my four-year-old son Ever's bedroom. And I thought he was in it.

...

On the heels of the Thomas Fire, which burned 282,000 acres over a period of several weeks in Ojai, Ventura, and Santa Barbara, California, came the Montecito mudslide of 2018. Nearly 200 million gallons of rainfall dropped in fifteen minutes in a record-breaking, middle-of-the-night storm, and the mountain gave way.

The mudslide killed twenty-three people. More than 150 people were injured, four of them critically. More than 450 homes and structures were damaged. A thirty-mile stretch of the 101 freeway was closed for almost a month because it was covered in several feet of slick, toxic mud that had to be cleared. A toddler and a teenage boy were never found. Destroyed cars had to be plucked from trees. Enormous boulders had to be jackhammered and removed. Houses, businesses, groves of protected oaks, and historical landmarks had to be dug out of the mud and restored. Many were lost forever. The beaches along the whole coast of Southern California were toxic and debris-covered for months. Full restoration of all the creeks and roads in Montecito would take two years; rebuilding and repairing the structures continue to this day. And my home was right at ground zero.

ACCEPTING THE INVITATION

Can you imagine that the worst thing that has ever happened to you might turn out to be a gift in disguise? Do you know that trauma, in whatever form it slayed you—childhood abuse, betrayal, divorce, the loss of a child, a diagnosis of terminal illness, a natural disaster—could be your initiation into a fuller, more illuminated and joyful life?

Trauma results from a moment, or a series of moments, in which we feel vulnerable, helpless, and weak; in which no escape seems possible; and in which, at some level, we are terrified we will not survive. This can happen even when our own safety is not directly at risk, but we are witnessing someone else's trauma. According to the US Substance Abuse and Mental Health Services Administration, trauma "results from an event, series of events, or set of circumstances experienced by an individual as physically or emotionally harmful or life-threatening with lasting adverse effects on the individual's functioning and mental, physical, emotional, or social well-being." To put it more simply and more inclusively, *trauma* is the Greek word for "injury." For our purposes, trauma is an event or injury that throws us off balance. An estimated 61 percent of men and 51 percent of women report having at least one traumatic event in their lifetimes.[1] These numbers are undoubtedly grossly under-representative because trauma includes all kinds of abuse, bullying, betrayal, near-death experiences, losses, combat or street violence, incest or rape, natural disasters, and pandemics.

Even as survivors carry with them the aftereffects of uncleared and unhealed trauma, many might not even recognize or define what has happened to them as traumatic. Some might know internally they were traumatized but don't feel safe to say so out loud. They might hold back because of shame (about sexual abuse, for instance), fear of repercussions or of being perceived as weak (as is common for men or for those traumatized in the line of duty), or lack of a safe person to tell.

I recognize that in the wake of trauma, during and sometimes even after healing, we can feel frustrated or even angry about considering the point of view that what we have suffered can lead anywhere good. It's okay if you don't feel that way yet. I've been there, and I empathize. Just know, if I've been there and can get here, so can you. It takes time, and it also takes healing.

As I sought my own healing, I found ways to heal from trauma thoughtfully and meaningfully, to return to harmonious well-being, and to find growth and resilience after a such an event. I found skillful and compassionate healers and guides, I discovered modalities proven by mainstream psychological and medical research, and I made leaps of faith with methodologies that at first seemed far-fetched but that sometimes led to profound posttraumatic growth.

In the weeks and months and years that followed the mudslide—although I was sometimes overcome with fear during bad weather, feelings of hopelessness that I would ever have my life "back together," and pain both physical and emotional—I also experienced blessings, growth, and depth I never could have imagined. My connection to prayer and manifesting desires became increasingly powerful. Gifts, literal and figurative, appeared. My relationships became stronger and deeper or fell away. Ultimately, my appreciation for life and my mission to enjoy it all and uplift others was fortified and crystallized. I chose to stride into this complex and growing field to find my way not only to surviving and being okay but to thriving, growing, and transcending. I began to write about my findings as a way to help others not only find their way back from trauma but transcend it.

The reality that the destruction of my world as I knew it would be a triumphant epiphany and invitation to live more rapturously and dynamically was a seed that would not be revealed for some time. I wrote this book to share how I transformed the darkness into light in order to encourage and ignite readers to break free from the heavy residue trauma can leave behind.

HOW TO USE THIS BOOK

In *Trusting the Dawn,* my hope is to offer tools, resources, and a framework for going through to come out the other side of trauma, to emerge transformed. This book is a companion for your journey from victimhood to initiation to a more dynamic and exalted life. I don't shy away from the realities of this path; it requires grit, toughness, vulnerability, and perseverance, and true healing takes longer than anyone wants it to. Ultimately, I seek to empower you not just to ask, "Why did this happen *to* me?" but also, "How did this happen *for* me?" Although the catalyst for this book was my acute traumatic experience, it is a call to action for everyone living in the modern age to see suffering as a call to identify, heal, and transmute trauma in order to appreciate the beauty of their lives.

With a bachelor's degree in English from Princeton University and a master's degree in clinical psychology from Pepperdine University, I had an intellectual understanding of the possibility for healing. My own transformative epiphanies outside of the classroom led me, along with my sister, Lucy, to found our company, Firestone Sisters, in 2012, with the aim of providing other people healing and growth opportunities. I have been producing and curating our Wild Precious Life Retreats for more than eight years and have led more than twenty retreats and workshops.

Through my own history and the stories of others I feature in this book, I found that trauma can crack open a new, intangible, rapturous, magical dimension of life that I never would have imagined was possible. There is potential for this kind of expansion through healing after the intense contraction of trauma. This dimension is always present, but our intellectual minds won't go there as long as we are safe, rested, coasting, and comfortable. As a result of experiencing extreme suffering—the loss of a loved one, a terminal illness, a near-death experience, any kind of abuse, the loss of a relationship or marriage, a betrayal—a sense of transparency between the physical world and the energetic/spiritual realms can become apparent. Through the initiatory experience of a traumatic event, life becomes more vivid and precious. This depth of power isn't something most of us can experience without the rawness and vulnerability of a crisis to drop us into it. As our rational intellect collapses, at least temporarily, we find greater ease in connecting to what lies beyond the physical limitations of the tangible world.

Trusting the Dawn combines my personal experience with input from experts ranging from medical doctors to mental health practitioners to alternative healers, and stories collected from other trauma survivors, along with information about the many avenues available for healing and renewal. The book is designed to engage and support you on a journey with others who've been through something similar and emerged transformed. Integrated throughout are my real-life stories along with in-depth interviews with other survivors.

In part 2, I share each healing practice I have come across and found helpful. For each modality, I'll provide a brief description and then get right to sharing the experiential part: the story of the way it was experienced, both during and afterward. I also provide suggestions for what you might do at home on your own or how to find a practitioner in your area and within your budget. (Where cost is an issue, don't be afraid to ask about sliding scales or pro bono sessions.) Additionally, I'll share whom each treatment might serve best and whether any should be avoided depending on your situation.

In the end, you will have the tools, resources, and encouragement to know you do not have to walk through the rest of your life permanently damaged or cursed. You do not have to be an eternal victim. You are, in fact, more complex, multidimensional, connected, and powerful *because* of what you have endured. My hope is that eventually and with healing you will recognize that trauma can be an incredible gift that yields wisdom and strength. This book provides revelatory inspiration, motivation, and tools to take healing to this next level, to empower you to know that you have the ability to alchemize great and lasting change.

For me, perhaps the biggest gift of trauma is recognizing the impermanence of this life and therefore valuing it. So often, we put off doing things we love, having important conversations, or spending time on what matters most to us. We punt our dreams to *next year*, or *when I have more money*, or *when I have a partner*. . . . Emerging from our darkest moments into the light teaches us that *now* is the only guarantee. It motivates and empowers us to seize the moment and live and love like we mean it.

PART 1

Transformation

WHY NOW?

The research and writing of this book began well before the Covid-19 pandemic, but what it offers became all the more relevant as billions of us entered into an indefinite period of lockdown, economic stress, and turmoil. Fear has erupted on a global scale, married to uncertainty about the future, which is sure to leave many with posttraumatic residue to heal and clear.

The aftermath of trauma can feel isolating. It might feel like it is hard for others to relate to what we're going through. Other people might distance themselves from us because they don't know how to be with us or what we need. Or on some subconscious (or conscious) level, they fear the trauma is "contagious." There could be shame surrounding the event that might cause us to retreat. There might be grief we want to process alone. We might feel we are the only one this has ever happened to, or certainly the only one we know of personally. Trauma is shocking; it can perpetuate fear and judgment, and it can cause others discomfort because it reminds us all that life is precious and fragile.

Considering our recent history with Covid-19, we are more isolated than ever. When we are kept from loved ones, schools, teachers, routines that offer us solace, people to connect with, support systems, and a sense of living life, these feelings of being alone are exacerbated. During this global crisis, the amount of trauma has increased. The collective fear alone is enough to make many of us, especially those of us who are more empathic, experience heightened anxiety. This communal fear can also be triggering for many of us with previous traumas. Domestic violence, sexual assault, divorce, depression, and suicide have all escalated during these periods of lockdown, uncertainty, and unrest.[1]

Sometimes, trauma is caused by systemic abuses such as racism or sexism, and those forms of abuse affect some people more than others. Those systemic problems are not resolved quickly. For those directly affected by them, the trauma might seem relentless and endless; how can healing begin when the wounds are continually inflicted? Although this is an absolutely crucial conversation to have, especially at this time in history, it is beyond the scope of this book.

One of the main reasons I wanted to write this book was to help you not to feel so alone. I know how alone I have felt at various times in my life while recovering from different traumatic events. And I recognize that I felt isolated even when I was surrounded by people who could and did help me and even while having access to resources and all of my physical needs met. Living in the United States on the East Coast until the age of twenty-five and the West Coast after that, I was in environments that for the most part supported the idea of therapy and healing. I had access to alternative healing modalities, and I continued to seek friends who shared my passion and desire for growth. Although affluence and access don't spare you from disaster or trauma, my support system and the nature of my trauma (the aftermath of a natural disaster is overt, and there is no shame or blame around it, unlike there can be with sexual abuse, for example) meant that I had immediate support from family and friends. We were also well insured, so we had assistance rebuilding our lives. Because of this, finding places to stay, clothes to wear, and eventually a new home to live in, as well as access to healing therapies was easier than it could have been. For those with different circumstances, the recovery from this kind of trauma can be a much harsher, longer journey.

I recognize how incredibly blessed I have been, and even so I still felt such shame, isolation, and hopelessness at times. I am writing this book for those of you who might not have the benefit of financial or emotional resources or who live somewhere where healing is discouraged, where you don't have access to the numerous healers and modalities available where I live. And also for those of you who, like me, have had the benefit of resources and access and still struggle. This book is an offering of healing resources and, ultimately, a community. I want you to know that you are not alone. You do not have to do this alone. You did nothing wrong. You are meant to grow and heal and live a joyful life full of love. Your hardest moments have provided you an opportunity for dynamic growth and contrast so that you can more fully appreciate all of the beauty, love, and goodness life has to offer you. What you have survived and are healing from has meaning. Your life has meaning.

This book and this community are here for you. You might be just beginning your healing journey by reading this book, or you might need some further inspiration and/or ideas on how to continue your metamorphosis. Wherever you are, this book is full of stories of other survivors, so you might find kindred spirits in these pages. There is no hierarchy of trauma. Each person's trauma is the worst because it happened to them. These pages are full of resources, tools, teachers, and practices to help you heal, thrive, and emerge resplendent.

With trauma being witnessed, identified, and named on an unprecedented scale in the world right now, healing work becomes even more urgent. Hurt people hurt more people unless they are healed; it is also true that hurt can be alchemized. As we do the work to heal and uplift ourselves, we help to heal and uplift others. There is a ripple effect in either direction: more hurt, anger, and fear or more love, acceptance, and unity. The world needs this kind of healing attention and love now more than ever. The time is now, and now is YOUR time. You are here. You are committed to your evolution. You are not alone.

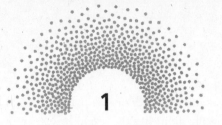

1

My Story

The months leading up to the Montecito mudslide of January 2018 had been unsettling for me. I felt almost crazy with uncertainty, so much so that I sought the advice of a psychic, something I had done only for fun before. I was desperately grasping for someone to tell me that everything was going to be okay. The Owl, as she called herself, made it even worse by telling me the coming months would be full of chaos. As she mused about why my soul had chosen this, I felt my internal panic bubble even higher.

My then husband, Napper, and I had recently bought a dreamy white farmhouse in Montecito. Our son had an enchanted oak forest to play in, and a baby sister was on the way. Old rose bushes pumped out fragrant, brightly hued blooms. We were just minutes from the celebrated Montecito Union public school, the beach, and Oprah Winfrey. What could go wrong with her as your neighbor? We were thrilled to be home.

And then, in early December, the Thomas Fire broke out. Newly pregnant, I was all for heeding the evacuation orders sent out as the sky went hazy gray-orange, the air became dangerous to breathe, and white ash dusted our cars and brick patio. We fled north to an Airbnb in Paso Robles and then eventually flew back east to ride out the seemingly endless season of this devastating fire. In early January 2018, the fire was mostly contained, so we returned home. We had only slept in the new house twice before the fire evacuation.

The night of the mudslide started out calm and almost balmy. A mandatory evacuation order went out because of forecasted rain, but it didn't include us. After dinner, I told Napper to put a couple of green moving bins in front of the doors in case any water might leak in. "Debris flow" sounded trivial. We weren't concerned.

As I got into bed for the fourth time in that bedroom, I had the overwhelming feeling that I really didn't like the room. It was, by all accounts, beautiful. It had been one of the home's main selling points. After reading a few pages of the intense book on karma for a spiritual book club my sister, Lucy, and I had formed with a few friends, I switched out the light and fell asleep.

For no reason that I am aware of, I woke up at 4 a.m. and jumped out of bed. We hadn't installed curtains in the bedroom, so I had a clear view of an orange glow up the hillside. It was one of the most eerily beautiful skies I'd ever seen, but far too early to be caused by the sunrise.

That glow turned out to be a massive gas line explosion. In its faint light, I saw the entire mountain coming at us. This tidal wave of mud, furniture, trees, and buildings was approaching our glass French doors at an incredible speed.

I screamed, "Oh my God, it's the mudslide! Get Ever!" Napper leapt out of bed and ran toward our son's room. I tried to follow him. I couldn't. Mud obliterated the doors and came crashing in. Mud up to my waist, filled with broken glass, pieces of furniture, rocks, branches. I had no choice. I had to turn around and run.

The sound of mud clearing a mountainside is deafening. (Most survivors of the mudslide continue to react strongly to loud noises.) Even as I ran for safety, I screamed for Napper and Ever, but no sound that came from me could make it past the sound of the world around me collapsing. Even as I watched the part of the house I thought contained my husband and son get swept away toward the ocean, I kept screaming for them.

Then, everything got quiet. The orangey pink light from the explosion up the hill didn't last long, but the sky did stay light long enough for me to see and assess the severity of the destruction all around me. In place of the trees and foliage that had surrounded our house were muddy heaps of rubble, a lone shoe, some dishes. My kitchen table had exploded out of the kitchen, the wall having given way as if it were cardboard; the table lay outside splintered in pieces, half buried in mud.

"Hello! Anybody there? Help! I need help!" I shouted from my perch on the bathroom countertop, with the mud, filth, and debris filling the room to the window, threatening the few free feet where I was crouched.

There was no response.

A neighbor's home was in view, but it was badly damaged, with mud sprayed all over the side and a caved-in wall. There were no signs of life outside my window.

From the orange clock that remained on the bathroom counter, I could see that it was about 5 a.m. when I was left in darkness on my tiny sliver of countertop, wet and cold with wintry rain, covered with mud from the waist down, and hunched in a ball, praying for the dawn to come so that I could see again.

I could feel myself dissociating, numbing out. My thoughts raced. *Please, oh please, let us be saved. Please let Napper and Ever be safe. Please let the baby in my belly be okay. Please let my family be okay. Maybe we should move to a remote island. Oh, but what about hurricanes?* I remembered reading that book on karma before falling asleep. *What is my karma, anyway, if this moment right now is where I ended up? Thank God I ate so much dessert last night; at least I'm not hungry.*

In the space between these racing thoughts, I experienced flashes that seemed like a dream of connection with something greater than myself and the physical world: soothing light, colors, and images that gave me the sense there was a loving presence with me. A window into the sacred opened just enough for me to peek through. These glimpses both calmed and thrilled me.

After hours of darkness, I saw a flashing light bouncing off the garage. I swung myself over the mud to the windowsill, squatted inside it, and yelled for help. I got a faint reply from a couple hundred yards away: "I'm from the fire department, but I can't get to you. I'll be back when it's light out." *When it's light out?!* Despair . . . and relief that someone knew I was alive and where I was as the hours ticked on.

And then, mercifully, dawn broke.

It wasn't a beautiful dawn. The harsh, steely light only revealed how truly stuck I was. I swung myself over the mud to the windowsill again and screamed for Napper and Ever. I tried not to imagine what could have happened.

And then, just as I started to swing back inside, I heard a faint "Babe? Mary?" Then, Ever's little voice: "Mommy? Mommy, where are you?"

It was the greatest relief I have ever known. *They were alive! We were all alive!* They sounded so far away. They'd had to creep out of their hideout in the upstairs bathroom to shout to me so I could hear them. Knowing they were so close and they were okay gave me a burst of hope, adrenaline, and will. Newly energized, I kept my mind busy by assessing and reassessing my surroundings, searching for a way out.

And then I started to smell gas.

As I worked on staying warm and lucid, I waited for the helicopters I had seen rescue neighbors from their rooftops return for me, my husband, and my child.

"Anybody here?"

I swung myself back to the windowsill. "I'm here! I'm here," I shouted.

A powerful and fearless-looking man was charging through the mud in waders. He hollered up to me, "We have to get you out of here."

I hesitated. "The helicopters will be back," I said.

He wasn't dressed in fire department regalia, and he had appeared as if from thin air. Who was this man? He told me his name was Orion. There was something so confident, calming, and brave about him; and let's face it, I wanted to get the hell out of there.

He said we couldn't wait. Who knew what could happen? It could start raining again, the gas might explode, the house might not hold. "Your husband and kid are okay. They've just been rescued," he told me.

"I thought they were dead," I heard myself say. Now that I knew it wasn't true, I had to say it out loud, to acknowledge what could have happened.

"I understand. My dad died in the La Conchita mudslide," Orion said matter of factly.

As he tried to figure out how to get me out of my frigid, muddy bathroom cell, I told him I was pregnant. This reinforced his determination to get me out without having me walk in the mud full of electrical wires, sewage, and broken glass. As the two of us searched for possible solutions, my panic started to rise at potentially being left again.

The door of the garage had collapsed inward, which allowed Orion to go inside and scour the wreckage. He wrested some surfboards from their hooks and placed them on top of the mud to create a makeshift bridge. After helping me out of the window, he steadied me while I balanced on the surfboards and walked away from my destroyed home.

A burly firefighter named Richard, dressed in a neon yellow jacket, waited for me where the mud and debris were a little shallower. Orion hoisted me onto Richard's back, and he carried me through the thick, slippery, thigh-high mud away from the house and up toward the crest of the hill, where I saw Napper and Ever waiting. The moment we were close enough to hug each other is one I will always remember in my heart and soul and every cell of my body.

•••

My near-death experience that night and believing for hours that my husband, son, and whole community might have been wiped out was a trauma on so many levels. It was as if all of the study of psychology and healing I had been doing my whole life had been meant to prepare me to survive it. Knowing it could have been so much worse—one or all of us could have died—heightened the impact of what we had been through.

Fast-forward to our exodus from a Federal Emergency Management Agency (FEMA) disaster zone in a six-wheeled National Guard truck. We sat in the truck, shoulder to shoulder with neighbors we were meeting for the first time under these mind-bending conditions. An older woman held Ever's hand as he sat on my lap. I tried to stop crying, to put on a brave face for Ever as he repeated the story of what had happened and asked, "Where are we going?" It pained me not to have any answers for him. We drove down one of the main arteries of Montecito, Coast Village Road, over trees and wreckage. A once bustling, affluent street had been transformed into apocalyptic ruins.

Seeing my cousin Andrew, ever positive and cheerful, part the crowd of refugees and volunteers to come scoop us up from the triage site in a supermarket parking lot, was one of the most relieving visions of my life. He had talked his way through police lines to pick us up and take us home with him. While we were in his truck on the way to his house, I happened to look back and see the most glorious double rainbow arcing over Montecito. So beautiful a sight in such a moment of devastation—maybe things were going to be all right.

Despite incredible love and support from family and friends, I had a paralyzing fear of the night. When I was lucky enough to fall asleep, I was ravaged by awful nightmares. A hot, unbearably itchy poison oak rash covered my legs where they had been plunged into the mud. When fear or nightmares didn't keep me up, the rash did.

Mostly, during this aftermath period, I felt like I was floating outside of my body. I wasn't really present. I kept striving to find the positive, the good, the light. If I let myself "go there," I feared I would never be able to heave myself out, and I had a preschooler to care for and a baby girl on the way. I had to stay in the light for them. I couldn't risk dropping into the depths I could feel roiling beneath the surface.

A few months later, I gave birth to a healthy baby girl, whom we named India Orion, for the hero who had saved us from the wreckage of our former home and life. These major life milestones forced me to be present in the moment, which delayed some of the trauma aftershocks until about a eighteen months later.

• • •

A year and a half after the mudslide, when I felt like life was getting back to normal, I had my first panic attack. Although I had done therapy sessions in the period directly following the mudslide—eye movement desensitization and reprocessing (EMDR), neurolinguistic programming (NLP), and cranial sacral therapy (CST)—and I had cleared a layer of the trauma, these panic attacks showed me there was more to excavate and clear.

On a hot fall day, my sister, Lucy, and I attended an outdoor event focused on introducing a new political candidate for county supervisor of Santa Barbara. We made small talk with neighbors about the heat, sipped sparkling water from sweating cans, and huddled in the shade of a sprawling avocado tree. As a celebrated actor (who had also lost his home in Montecito during the mudslide) began his introduction of the candidate, I found a spot in the shade where I could see. After the introduction, the candidate began her campaign speech. I was nodding and smiling, feeling just fine as she railed against the cannabis industry. Then, she moved to her next talking point about natural disasters and mudslides. She pointed out that it wasn't a matter of *whether* they would happen again but *when*.

I had the thought, "Oh! Everyone is going to look at me to see how I'm doing with this mudslide talk." And then I felt myself slipping toward a full faint. I started sweating a lot, and not because of the heat. I ducked from under the tree branches, weaving my way over to Lucy and out of the crowd.

"I think I'm going to faint," I managed to whisper to Lucy.

She followed me to some plastic lawn chairs. I collapsed into one of them next to an old woman who didn't bat an eyelash. My vision blurred. My clothing was wet with sweat. I lost control of my body and was barely conscious. Lucy kept urging me to walk out to the driveway or at least the sidewalk, but I couldn't even stand. Finally, she got me to the driveway, where I collapsed on the ground.

A stranger brought me a glass of water. Some friends ushered over a doctor who checked my pulse and my pupils, asked me some questions, and told me I'd be fine with a little rest. I went home and laid down, and as I recovered, I tried to figure out what was wrong with me. *Had I eaten something bad? Did I have a bug?* I didn't identify this event as a panic attack until something clicked a week or so later. My suspicion that this was what happened was confirmed when I experienced my second panic attack in the midst of a nonprofit luncheon honoring incredible therapeutic work for children in underserved communities.

Just hearing someone speak about how damaging trauma can be set my heart racing, my whole body sweating, and my head spinning. That's when

I realized how much more healing I had to do. I was so far from okay. I had excavated a layer of trauma, or maybe two, but there were many more layers to go. I was just at the beginning.

And so, I recommitted to the path of healing as completely and profoundly as possible, for myself and for my family—and as an offering to others haunted by traumas they have physically survived. This book is that offering. Through healing we can free ourselves.

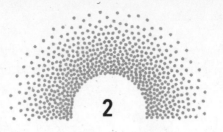

The Mind, Heart, and Body in Trauma

So much has been written about the damaging (and damning) effects of trauma on the body and the brain. As I researched for both myself and this book, I found that reading about all of the possibilities, symptoms, and residue trauma *can* leave behind was, frankly, traumatizing! Just as many first-year medical students imagine themselves afflicted with each new disorder and disease they study, I was searching myself for manifestations of the variety of symptoms described. The power of suggestion is considerable. Given that we are all unique in our biology as well as in how we distinctively process even the same trauma, I have found the generalization of symptoms and scenarios belittling and even infuriating. This is especially true because the assumptions made usually undermine survivors by forecasting a far-from-ideal outcome for them/us. I also recognize that for some, a diagnosis is validating and helps to design an effective treatment plan.

Psychology is a young science and is evolving all the time. The *Diagnostic and Statistical Manual of Mental Disorders*, fifth edition (DSM-5), sometimes referred to as the bible of psychiatric diagnoses, has been updated and revised to remove, add, and amend diagnoses several times since its initial publication in 1952.[1] Because my book is an offering for you to heal and thus feel lighter, more empowered, and free from trauma, I am going to keep the discussion on all of the possible effects of trauma brief. If you want to delve deeper, I recommend Bessel van der Kolk's books on trauma.

THE PHYSICAL

Our brains and bodies are ingeniously designed to survive and thrive. One way we do this is to effectively respond to danger. When we perceive a threat, our bodies go into freeze, fight, or flight mode. We assess whether it is best to freeze, making ourselves hard to detect; fight, warding off an assailant; or take flight as quickly as possible. When we are in this state of heightened arousal, the sympathetic nervous system—the one responsible for this fight-or-flight response—is activated, releasing adrenaline and cortisol, allowing us to focus while also shunting blood away from our organs to our extremities so we are better able to outrun the perceived threat or fight it. Our senses are heightened in this state of hypervigilance so that we can best navigate the danger and keep ourselves safe.

This function is healthy and a key factor in our survival. Issues arise when the trauma from the incident is not discharged and released after we are safe. The chemicals that help us get to safety can remain stored in the body and brain. Excess amounts of adrenaline and cortisol in the body can tax our adrenal glands, leaving us exhausted and in a state of perpetual hypervigilance. In this state we startle more easily, we are more reactive to stimuli, and we can be jumpy and irritable.

Digestion

Board-certified structural integration practitioner Lauren Roxburgh, dubbed the "Body Whisperer," explains that held trauma can result in weight gain. The body, thinking it is still under threat because of elevated cortisol levels, retains calories as a way of protecting itself from starvation and/or impact. Furthermore, as I previously mentioned, one of the features of the body switching into fight-or-flight mode is diverting blood from the organs and functions such as digestion so that more energy is available to run from a threat or fight it. Therefore, our digestion can be disrupted and inharmonious if we are holding on to trauma.

While healing, try eating cooked, soothing foods, such as soups and stews, that don't require a lot of effort to digest. Avoid raw vegetables, fruits, and salads until your digestion regulates. Excessive alcohol, caffeine, and processed foods can also exacerbate digestion issues.

Sleep

Because of the state of hyperarousal that can linger after a traumatic event, sleep might be disturbed or peppered with nightmares. I know this was true for me. I have been a good sleeper for most of my life, but after the mudslide I found myself struggling to go to sleep and then awakening because of nightmares throughout the night. Nightmares typically plague about 72 percent of people in the wake of trauma. Unfortunately, the nightmares can make it hard to go back to sleep, which in turn leads to fatigue, which can exacerbate other symptoms.[2] At night, I was afraid of sounds, trees falling and collapsing the roof, a tidal wave surging up and through the house, an intruder, you name it! If it was terrifying, my mind imagined it. And that was *before* I managed to fall asleep. If I did sleep, flashback-like nightmares kept waking me.

Neuroscientists understand that rapid eye movement (REM) is the sleep cycle most affected after a traumatic event.[3] This makes sense because REM is the deepest and most restorative sleep, when we dream. What I find fascinating is that after my first EMDR session (see chapter 7), a treatment modality that mimics this REM cycle, my nightmares abruptly stopped. During REM sleep, your eyes move back and forth, and EMDR simulates this by stimulating that bilateral movement. Because we are all unique human beings, there is no guarantee that EMDR will end nightmares, but for me, the relief was profound.

It also helps to feel safe when you sleep. Keep a phone nearby and a loved one who lives close by on alert. If you can and it is appropriate, have someone sleep with you. There was a period after the mudslide when Ever wanted to sleep in the bed with me after having been an independent sleeper. And then there was a time when I wanted him to sleep in the bed with me. This only lasted for about a week but was comforting to us both.

Try taking a warm bath containing lavender before bed. Read only pleasant stories before bed. If you become incredibly restless in bed, after about twenty minutes get up, read something soothing, journal, meditate, and then when you feel more relaxed get back into bed.

If your sleep is more significantly disturbed, it might be worth exploring imagery rehearsal therapy (IRT), invented in 1978 by Isaac Marks. Through rewriting the scripts of recurrent nightmares so that they are no longer terrifying, and rehearsing these new scripts during the day, you can alleviate the nightmares. A study conducted with survivors of sexual assault practicing IRT found a 60 percent reduction of disturbing dreams and correlating symptoms of posttraumatic stress disorder (PTSD). Another tool to potentially discuss with your doctor for alleviating extreme nightmares and sleep disturbances is the pharmaceutical prazosin. Prazosin is a beta-blocker, which means that it attaches to the fear receptors in the brain, decreasing their response. It first came on the market in the 1970s as a means to lower blood pressure. The added benefit of prazosin in decreasing dreaming and therefore alleviating nightmares was discovered later.[4]

THE EMOTIONAL

When we experience a trauma, our amygdala, the part of our brain responsible for managing emotional memories, becomes activated and may associate contextual surroundings and situations with the trauma. These objects, places, scents, tastes, sounds, and feelings can act as triggers afterward, although they seem completely unrelated. For me, during the mudslide, an inordinate amount of mud surrounded me, keeping me trapped and threatening to carry me away to my death. For months following the mudslide, the smell of earthy mud, even in a calm and lovely setting, while hiking or using a mud mask on my face, would trigger a fear response. My amygdala had connected the smell of mud with danger, indicating that I still had more healing to do. Although this hypervigilance can be annoying at best and paralyzing at worst, it can also be helpful in terms of indicating more we have to release and heal.

When danger presents itself, the amygdala alerts the brainstem, which activates our freeze, fight, or flight response. Usually the amygdala remains more vigilant for about ninety days following a traumatic event, although it can get stuck in the "on" position, which can lead us to experience higher anxiety levels or even panic attacks.

THE SPIRITUAL

According to shamanism and ancient mystical systems, when a trauma occurs the spirit can be shocked out of the body. There is a separation between body and soul. In a sense, the soul might ascend to a higher dimension, where there is support and divine guidance. This serves to spare the brain and body greater suffering. It's as if our soul goes in search of what will allow us our most fulfilling, comforting, dynamic way through and forward.

COMMUNAL TRAUMA

Currently we are enduring communal trauma in the wake of the Covid-19 pandemic, which has affected all of us in one way or another. I also experienced communal trauma after September 11, 2001 (9/11) while living in New York City, and then again more directly in the Montecito mudslide. I have noticed that when trauma occurs on the communal level, people come together. Friends, family, neighbors, and strangers step up to help and to support each other.

Edith Eger, a Holocaust survivor and bestselling author with a thriving clinical psychology practice in La Jolla, California, shares in her book *The Gift* how communal trauma can be easier to relinquish when it is acknowledged, accepted, and accounted for within the collective. "It's easier to release the past when others see your truth, tell the truth. When there's a collective process—restorative justice, war crimes tribunals, truth and reconciliation committees—through which perpetrators are accountable for the harm they inflicted, and the court of the world holds the truth to the light."[5]

William James, a well-respected historian, psychologist, and philosopher who taught at Harvard and Stanford Universities, wrote a lot about communal trauma in the aftermath of the San Francisco earthquake of 1906. James, at Stanford when the earthquake struck, put the experience of resilience and community into words: "I now know fully what I have always believed, that the pathetic way of feeling great disasters belongs rather to the point of view of the people at a distance than to the immediate victims. I heard not a single really pathetic or sentimental word in California expressed by anyone."[6] He remarked upon and recorded the sense of fellowship, initiative, orderliness, helpfulness, and awakening that occurred in the people of San Francisco following the earthquake.

I noticed this too after the mudslide. A civilian bravely rescued me, strangers offered water and snacks at the triage site, and friends and strangers found us housing, clothing, support, and anything else we might have needed. In her book on communal traumas, Rebecca Solnit concludes:

> Many fear that in disaster we become something other than what we are—helpless or bestial and savage in the most common myths— or that is who we really are when the superstructure of society crumbles. We remain ourselves for the most part, but freed to act on, most often not the worst but the best within. The ruts and routines of ordinary life [which get eclipsed in disasters/traumas] hide more beauty than brutality.[7]

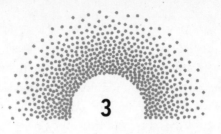

3

The Reframe,
and Why Now?

Trauma has become an important topic in modern life. This is the era in which a pandemic, racial injustice, economic inequality, and the MeToo movement are part of everyday conversation. Trauma is moving from the shadows to the forefront to be addressed, and its role in creating many of the problems that individuals and societies face is increasingly well understood. None of us gets through life without being traumatized in one way or another. As spiritual teacher and bestselling author Gabby Bernstein shared in an interview with Lewis Howes on his podcast *The School of Greatness,*

> We're all traumatized—everybody. Everyone that's walking through this world, every human being, they may not have had trauma like we've had, but they're walking through life feeling unsafe. It's in these subtle moments, as *A Course in Miracles* says, "the moments that we detour into fear they call the descent from magnitude into littleness. And we then create this form of ego, which is a separate mind, separate from God, separate from love, separate from freedom, and it builds up a pretense around us."

At the root of much posttraumatic residue is this feeling of separateness, both within the self and in the world. The traumatic incident becomes a fragment within us until we heal and integrate it. In relation to the outside world, we can feel as if we are the only ones who have experienced such terror, pain, and suffering. If we can find our way to healing, integration of the event(s), and ultimately a sense of wholeness both internally and with the world, we can recalibrate and let go of our trauma by recognizing it as a part of us and humanity.

Trauma can also make us idealize the "normal from before" or imagine that life, love, and happiness exist somewhere else outside of us. Bestselling author, cancer survivor, and spiritual teacher Mark Nepo eloquently expresses this: "We either willfully shed or are broken open. One of the hardest things is to accept what is. When we're broken open there is an acceptance that we have to work with what is. The only way out is through. What's in the way is the way." We must go toward and get underneath the pain of loss, betrayal, and trauma so we can "remake the maps of a landscape that has been blown up. The old maps are obsolete." Nepo reminds us in my interview with him, "Great love and great suffering show us that the miracle of life is wherever we are. Great love and great suffering bring us to our knees and show us that it's all right here. It's always been right here."

The human experience involves suffering at times. And there is no hierarchy of suffering. Each person's suffering is the most intense for them. Each person's challenge is part of their unique evolution. To compare our pain and suffering to another's would either diminish or inflate our own, distorting our experience in either direction. My hope with this book is that you will not compare your trauma to mine or the other trauma stories told here but be inspired that if we could overcome it, so can you.

The ultimate purpose of this book is for trauma to be reframed as an opportunity and healed, and for true transformation and thriving to be possible in its aftermath. Nepo emphasizes, "It's not to try and reframe things in a Pollyanna way. Do I want the suffering of it, no. It's always hard when in it to appreciate whatever lesson is going to come from it. That's at the heart of faith. I'm seldom grateful when I'm struggling, but faith is knowing that I will be." Getting to the point where this reframe feels authentic is a process most people navigate in the same way a character in John Green's novel *The Fault in Our Stars* experienced falling in love: "*slowly, and then all at once.*" It might initially provoke anger or frustration to imagine that the worst thing that's ever happened to us can also be an opportunity.

This does not mean growth occurs without any kind of distress; often they coexist.[1] As L. G. Calhoun and R. G. Tedeschi, psychologists and professors who study posttraumatic growth, explain, just as an earthquake can alter the physical environment, a trauma, because of its "unusual, uncontrollable, potentially irreversible, and threatening qualities," can shift how we perceive the world and make sense of it. There can be a new and more urgent way to find meaning in life. The reassessment and revaluation of life plant "seeds for new perspectives and a sense that valuable—although painful—lessons have been learned."[2]

RESILIENCE AND EXPANSION

Although there is much focus on the negative impact of trauma, studies have investigated how trauma, when healed and integrated, can in fact make us more resilient and dynamic. Michael Rutter of King's College in London, referred to as "the father of child psychology," has focused much of his career on resilience. In 2006, Rutter defined resilience as "an interactive concept that is concerned with the combination of serious risk experiences and a relatively positive psychological outcome despite those experiences." In 2012, Rutter came up with the term *resilience theory* when he discovered that monkeys separated from their mother for two hours daily, which caused them trauma, appeared to manage later stress significantly better than those monkeys who did not have that experience.[3] Rutter describes this as a "steeling (or strengthening) effect."[4] The possibility for greater tolerance for stress as well as increased plasticity in the brain can result from enduring adversity. In other words, science has proven that exposure to stressful situations can in fact make you more resilient, stronger, and better able to deal with and manage future challenges. Good news indeed.

Research shows that experiences of growth following a traumatic event are far more likely than posttraumatic stress disorder (PTSD).[5] But healing, integrating, and reframing our traumatic experiences becomes even more important because there is also evidence that unhealed trauma can create genetic changes that can be passed down through generations. This also means that if you have a parent, grandparent, or ancestor who didn't heal a serious trauma, you might be genetically predisposed to having a heightened response to a threatening experience.[6] Knowing that my healing directly affects my children, and frankly anyone who comes into contact with me, is a motivating reason to continue on the healing path.

Many trauma survivors experience growth and expansion in their lives, such as "improved relationships, new possibilities for one's life, a greater appreciation for life, a greater sense of personal strength and spiritual development. There appears to be a basic paradox apprehended by trauma survivors who report these aspects of posttraumatic growth: Their losses have produced valuable gains."[7] Perhaps this paradox induces feelings of guilt or even a sense of disbelief that such positive outcomes could be born of something so tragic. But placing expectations and projections upon survivors to be "happy" doesn't leave much room for individual experiences and expressions of positive outcomes. Does it seem improper? Too fast? Too joyful? For what and to whom are we holding ourselves and our own precious evolution accountable?

This reframe can begin with a confluence of approaches. Healing therapies I present and explore in detail in later chapters are, of course, pivotal to the release and reconfiguration of trauma. To set the stage for these therapies to be most effective, shifting our language and thinking makes for the most fertile healing ground.

LANGUAGE

We use language all day long, every day, whether we think it, write it, or speak it. The power of our words isn't often considered. In ancient Celtic and other Anglo-Saxon cultures, the spoken and written word were considered magical, in the sense of weaving a spell. This belief is the origin of the word *spelling*.

Subtle shifts in our language are available to us all in each and every moment, particularly around a traumatic event and ourselves. Begin to notice the story you are telling yourself—how are you speaking to yourself? There can be a familiar traumatic story loop akin to: "After the event, my life was over. I was such a bright, happy person and then this ruined my life." Although there is significance in speaking the story while moving through the shock, anger, and grief, if we don't move beyond this point, we allow the trauma to color our present and future despite the fact that it occurred in the past. Staying in this place leaves you in a perpetual trauma loop, and the trauma is continuing to emanate from YOU.

Is your internal dialogue one of blame and excuses? Are you present in your daily life or giving your power away to events of the past or a future out of reach? What did you learn about yourself, gain access to in yourself, come to understand because of what you survived that made you a more multi-dimensional, faceted, capable person? As James Gordon, a Harvard-trained trauma expert with more than forty years in the field, says, "Trauma is the soil from which wisdom and compassion grow."

- **Consider Your Narrative:** Considering that our thoughts, ultimately made up of words, shape and create our reality, being impeccable with our words is the difference between a desired existence and an undesirable one. Become conscious of where you are focusing your attention and how the mere fact of focusing on what you *do* desire brings more of that into your life. And be aware that a thought like "I don't want to be depressed" is focused on feeling depressed. Alternatively, "I give thanks for feeling joyful" is a positive statement for what you desire. Giving thanks as if this state already exists tricks the brain into believing that it does.

- **Show Up for Yourself:** Be mindful about how you speak to yourself about yourself. Do you cancel on yourself? Tell yourself you're going to do something and not do it? When we do that, we are teaching ourselves we're not worth showing up for, and our words are empty and not believable. If we don't honor ourselves, why would we expect others to honor us? It's helpful to think again about how you would speak to a friend or someone you care about. Often, we are much harsher with ourselves than we are with others.

- **Speak in Third Person:** Srini Pillay, a Harvard-trained psychiatrist who coaches others on leading more dynamic lives, suggests in an interview with Anna Cabeca that speaking to ourselves in the third person is actually more effective. For example, I would say, "*Mary* is going to rock this" rather than "*I* am going to rock this."

- **Banish the Not:** Pillay also asserts that when we use the word "not," our brain doesn't register it and simply hears the rest of it. "I will not get upset" translates to us getting upset. Instead, saying "I will remain calm" is more effective.

Edith Eger is a Hungarian-born survivor of Auschwitz who went on to become a prolific author and psychologist living in La Jolla, California. She has helped and inspired many people who have suffered trauma. In her memoir, *The Choice*, she expounds on the idea that we all choose the role in which we cast ourselves in our own stories. She writes,

> Suffering is universal. But victimhood is optional. We are all likely to be victimized in some way in the course of our lives. At some point we will suffer some kind of affliction or calamity or abuse, caused by circumstances or people or institutions over which we have little or no control. This is life. And this is victimization. It comes from the outside. In contrast, victimhood comes from the inside. No one can make you a victim but you. We become victims not because of what happens to us but when we choose to hold on to our victimization. We develop a victim's mind—a way of thinking and being that is rigid, blaming, pessimistic, stuck in the past, unforgiving, punitive, and without healthy limits or boundaries. We become our own jailors when we choose the confines of the victim's mind.[8]

So many of us, myself included, allow our traumas to take on an amplified and inflated role in our life stories, the stories we tell ourselves and other people; we allow them to define us. Pillay says that continuing to tell the story "cements the memory and keeps the suffering online."[9] So much of my story, *for twenty years,* was: "I was molested several times in childhood." There were stories around the story, and it wound up becoming a big, heavy load I was toting around with me.

Although we don't want to get stuck in a negative story loop or in any way let a story of trauma define who we are, there is incredible power in speaking your truth and sharing your story, especially if the purpose is to help others (here's a whole book about it!). We have witnessed the power of speaking up for ourselves through the Black Lives Matter movement, the MeToo movement, and Take Back the Night, a nonprofit organization that has held events since 1976 for sexual abuse survivors to share their stories. I am by no means suggesting we don't share our stories of trauma by speaking them out loud so that we may heal, hold others accountable, and open up safe space for others to share their truths. I am suggesting we reconsider how and when and how often we tell those stories. Several of the survivors and thrivers I interviewed for this book referred me to other sources for the details of their traumas, preferring not to put themselves through it again by recounting it step by step. They were much more focused on the healing part of their stories, how they had alchemized the darkness into something brilliant.

My story about childhood abuses led to some positive outcomes, such as the deep healing path I found myself on and offered to others through the retreats I produce. As I huddled on the bathroom counter during the mudslide, I gave thanks for the healing I had done thus far and for some of the tools I had acquired that I put to use in the moment and then afterward. I was putting Rutter's resilience theory to the test! Had previous, though entirely different, trauma made me more resilient and able to handle and recover from this new one?

And then there was the new story. It started as "I almost died in the Montecito mudslide." Over time, with conscious energy, thought, and help from healers, I shifted it from that version, which kept me in the victim role of something happening *to* me, to "I survived the mudslide." A slight shift, and yet it transforms me from playing the passive victim role of almost dying to the active role of surviving. I remember being so indignant when a French healer reeking of cigarettes told me in her heavily accented English, "Just get over it. Leave it behind. It is done! It is over!" I thought, *If it were that easy, why would I be here? Why wouldn't I just do that?* And yet, she had a point that we can get stuck in thought loops and let the story define us; she just could have delivered it better!

There is something so freeing and healing about not defining yourself by the negative events that have happened in your life. Yes, they proved that you were fierce and brave and resilient and even a little bit magical, so let that be the story. Don't get into the gory details of your trauma when introducing yourself because that can actually be retriggering and retraumatizing. Before thinking about what you are sending out into the world, let's focus on your internal world and the story you tell yourself about yourself.

. . . .

EXERCISE: REWRITING YOUR STORY

Experiment with adjusting your story to one of triumphant surviv-al. Of resilience, of perseverance. Of uncovering beautiful, strong, more compassionate aspects of yourself and your life by having gone through and come out the other side. You are strong. You are resilient. You are meant to be here. You are meant to shine your light more brightly and more fully. You are playing a part in alchemizing the darkness to become light. You are brave. You are loved. The very fact that you are reading this book means that you are already in an alchemical state where the darkness and hurt that permeated your trauma is transforming. You are in the process of becoming more than you were before. You are in a state of opening your heart, of expansion, in which so much more love and beauty is possible, for yourself and others. How did you/do you exhibit these characteristics? Journal it or speak it out loud, and reframe your own story. For me, the focus in rewriting my story was on shifting the narrative from "I almost died. My son and husband almost died. My mother would have died if she were sleeping in my guest house as planned" to "I survived. My loved ones survived. I woke up in time; I was safe. I was divinely protected. It was not my time, and I am meant to be here to thrive and help others." Work on shifting your story to one that casts you in the role of active survivor rather than passive victim.

ACCEPTANCE AND FORGIVENESS

Acceptance is a key piece in integrating trauma. Through integration, allowing all of our experiences to be part of who we are, we become whole. When we are whole, we are empowered, and transformation and evolution can transpire. Fully accepting the event(s) doesn't have to mean forgiving the person or circumstance that hurt you if that is too much of a stretch for you at this moment, but accepting what occurred means we don't have it stuffed away. We are fully aware of it so that it doesn't have to remain in a dark corner, ultimately keeping us in that place. The idea is that your acceptance and forgiveness is ultimately for *you,* not for the cause of the trauma. Eger, the Holocaust survivor, shared this perspective in our interview:

There is no forgiveness without rage. You go through the valley of the shadow of death, but you don't camp there, you go through it. And you refuse to be the victim. It's not your identity. It's not who you are. It's what was done to you. And you don't minimize it, you don't run from it or fight it. It's what I call my cherished wound. Auschwitz was my opportunity to discover that life is inside out.

No one makes me happy. I make me happy. I am in total charge
of my thinking, feeling, and behaviors.

I had grappled for a lifetime with not having forgiven the seventy-year-old
man who molested my seven-year-old self. The perpetrator was long gone,
having died decades ago, yet I was still alive and was less free and loving because I had not forgiven him. Some part of me recognized that I continued
to hurt myself by not allowing my forgiveness to unfold. What finally helped
me to forgive and release him and that trauma was beginning to understand
what must have happened to him as a child that would in turn have him act
that out with me. It isn't easy and took me years, and sometimes I still feel
my resentment creep in, but for me, acknowledging it and sending the child
version of that seventy-year-old man forgiveness, helps me live and love
more freely. Living with resentment only causes us more pain and suffering.
In fact, resentment can fester into disease in the body if left unchecked and
uncleared. Acceptance, and taking responsibility for our response to what
has happened in our lives, puts us in an empowered, active position rather
than the passive one of victim.

Another concept that top spiritual teachers, including Deepak Chopra,
Don Miguel Ruíz, and Gabby Bernstein, impart is taking full responsibility for everything in your life. That means *everything*. I wondered how
I could have been responsible for being molested as a child. This doesn't
mean blaming ourselves, thinking we actively did something to cause it,
or seeing ourselves as diminished in any way. The adults those children
become can take responsibility to seek the right help and, through the
experience of healing, further their evolution.

Martin grew up in low-income neighborhoods where abuse, addiction,
and gang violence were the norm. He spent his formative years in and out
of juvenile hall and jail. The traumas he endured that landed him there,
and the trauma he experienced while incarcerated, eventually found an
outlet in the form of healing through connection with elders and sweat
lodge rituals based in his Native American roots.

A key piece in his healing was accepting responsibility for his actions while
also holding others accountable. Martin made a promise to be of service, which
took shape when he discovered his passion for education (he has a bachelor's
degree in psychology and a master's degree in sociology and is working on his
doctoral degree in education). He leads by example, actively participating in
educating at-risk youth, showing them there is another, better way.

Martin credits daily spiritual work (he spends time in nature every day), keeping a safe distance from certain friends and family members still acting out behaviors and emotions of the past, and connection with elders as the most healing behaviors in his life. He also acknowledges that in his own healing, he is healing generational trauma. He's healing his ancestors and also healing his daughter and those who come after him. Martin says that this self-actualization work has led to feeling peace of mind, to being comfortable in his own skin. It has been a "journey to myself" that he doesn't want to end.

Nepo shares in our interview,

> I struggle; I think some things are unforgivable, like genocide and the Holocaust. My understanding of forgiveness so far goes back to the meaning of the word, which literally means "to give for," so it's an exchange. An exchange for what? For me forgiveness is not about the other person; when I'm wounded, part of my heart is preoccupied, it is not available to live life. So forgiveness is really exchanging the wounded part of my heart in an earned way, not in a "that was fine" sort of way, so that I can regain the wholeness of my heart to live my life.

FOCUS

Our words and thoughts have such power in creating our experiences. Becoming conscious of where we focus our attention, and how the mere fact of focusing on what we *do* desire brings more of that into our lives, is an essential step. Interestingly, most of us spend a lot of our energy focusing on what we don't want! A thought like "I want more money" is focused on the lack of wealth. Alternatively, "I give thanks for all of the abundance in my life" is a positive statement for what you desire. Giving thanks as if the abundance already exists tricks the brain into believing that it is already so. Note that the intention is not only to think/write/speak the words but also to link those statements to the positive feeling the words elicit. Gratitude is an excellent way out of the crushing feelings of PTSD. Several studies have shown that actively practicing gratitude wards off symptoms of PTSD and results in a better quality of life.

OUR ENVIRONMENT

Another important factor in effective healing is raising our awareness about the people, events, and media we allow into our space. Be fierce about who you spend time with, choosing to be around those who lift you up and make you feel good. As you do more of this work, heal, and become more conscious, you will begin to notice more how you feel when you are with others. It can be confusing at first to even identify which feelings belong to you and which you are observing and picking up from those around you.

With practice, you will actively *feel* if people are not in energetic alignment with themselves and you. Certain relationships make us feel warm, happy, optimistic, loving, and safe. Other times, we might spend time with someone who makes us feel sad, heavy, or anxious, and when we leave them, we feel drained. Start to notice the people and places that make you feel good, and begin to allow yourself more time and space for them while implementing firm boundaries with those in your life who make you feel worse. This includes family! Family can often have the most heartwarming, supportive energy, but familial ties can also be fraught with historic or even ancestral unhealed trauma. It is okay (and in some cases, imperative to your well-being) to have firm boundaries with such family members.

It's also important to be aware of your physical surroundings. After determining they are safe, make sure you are spending your time in a soothing environment that feels good to you. Hanging inspiring and beautiful artwork, buying a potted plant or fresh flowers, painting a wall your favorite color, and keeping your space clean and organized are all ways your external environment can help you maintain a tranquil inner environment. Be aware of your work space as well. Most of us spend a lot of our time at work, so as much as possible, work with positive people in an environment that feels good.

Be disciplined about your news intake and engagement on social media. The news is full of stories that trigger you on a primal level: fear. Select a few news outlets that are as unbiased as possible, and check in with them on a schedule, never first thing in the morning or before going to bed. Also, be mindful of the kind of entertainment you watch, read, and listen to. Avoid programming that spikes your adrenaline (thrillers, murder mysteries, etc.). As with relationships, if you notice you feel badly while watching/reading/listening to something, change the channel!

• • • •

EXERCISE: GRATITUDE

A good exercise for moving toward forgiveness is practicing gratitude. By adjusting our focus to what we have in our lives, we are
reminded of why we want to be here and thriving. Write down
three things you are grateful for; they can be as simple as "my health,
my morning coffee, flowers, the ocean, my children," and so forth.

USING YOUR VOICE

The ability to express ourselves can be oppressed during and after trauma.
We might have been unable to speak or scream during a traumatic event,
and we might also have been silenced afterward. Either it felt too scary or
shameful to speak about what happened, or we were told to keep quiet.
Regardless of whether it was conscious, so many of us have received a message that it was unsafe to use our voices and to be heard.

While writing this book I grappled with fears of being judged for myriad
reasons. I go deep into the concept of past lives further in the book, but as a brief
introduction, many cultures acknowledge and understand that we as beings re-
incarnate. Science also has shown that energy can't be created or destroyed, and
if we are all energy, what happens to that energy when our bodies die? Again, I
explain more in the section on past life regression later in the book. One profound fear manifested for me repeatedly in images of my being killed for helping
and healing others. Whether I was envisioning past lives in which I was a healer
burned at the stake for being a "witch" or whether it was just my current fears
presenting themselves in that way, the fear was real. Yet through these images,
many of my current fears abated. I had this understanding: *Oh, no wonder I'm
afraid. I got killed for this before. Whatever happens this time, I am not going to die
for speaking my truth and shining a light into the darkness.*

When we speak up, we become more visible, and we might incur
judgment. A therapist once said to me that people are judging all of us
all the time anyway, so go ahead and do what you want to do! Speak up,
take the path you really want to take, end that relationship, go for that
job, be true to yourself. If you are in an abusive relationship or live in
a culture that is acutely dangerous, speak your truth to people who can
help you, not to those who could harm you.

Also, in my experience, you speaking your truth and expressing yourself gives others permission to do the same. And that helps us all understand each other, connect more honestly and deeply, and know we are not alone and are seen and heard.

THE WHOLE YOU

Integration, meaning assimilating and bringing together aspects of your experience that might feel separate, is key to healing. When we are traumatized, we have a natural and at first healthy instinct to push away that experience and any feelings and sensations associated with it. In self-preservation, we distance ourselves from that experience, understandably, because we want to get on with our lives, feel better, and not dwell on something that caused us pain.

Richard Schwartz, who invented internal family systems (IFS) therapy, identified that we all have different parts within ourselves. All of us. When we become traumatized, though, certain parts of ourselves present at the time of the trauma might get stuck in a negative loop about it. Some of these parts continue to exhibit behaviors that were adaptive and helpful at the time of the trauma but have outlived their usefulness. When these behaviors become maladaptive, and we repeat them to get away from a perceived threat when there is no threat, we are showing symptoms of PTSD. As a way to move past these behaviors and symptoms, IFS therapy works with the various parts of the self to understand them, empower them, and allow them to integrate with the whole. Schwartz refers to the youngest traumatized parts of ourselves as "the exiles." They might feel unable to stop judging the situation or helpless to protect us or remain hypervigilant about that trauma repeating itself. Schwartz found that "when the clients' parts felt safe and were allowed to relax, the clients would experience spontaneously the qualities of confidence, openness, and compassion that [he] came to call the Self. [He] found that when in that state of Self, clients would know how to heal their parts."[10]

It would seem the goal of working with all of our parts, allowing them to feel seen, safe, and relaxed, is to be whole: to accept and ultimately appreciate and love all of the aspects of ourselves so there is no internal struggle between them. And then all the roles we play are in alignment, working together harmoniously and with integrity.

This concept of integration comes up again and again throughout various modalities. Trauma expert and therapist Pat Ogden, founder of the

Sensorimotor Psychotherapy Institute, went as far as to say that integration is always the goal of trauma therapy. She explains that often trauma happens too fast and is too overwhelming for it to be integrated in the moment. Ogden shared what Onno van der Hart, one of her friends and colleagues, calls trauma-related dissociation, in which part of us is still living in "trauma time," as if the event is still happening, so therefore it is not integrated.

Ultimately, if parts of our past, bodily sensations, and aspects of ourselves are pushed aside, ignored, or discounted, there will be tension within us. We will be at war with ourselves. By acknowledging, accepting, forgiving, honoring, and eventually loving all of these parts of ourselves and our history, we become whole. In becoming whole, we feel peace, love, and harmony.

INITIATION

After the mudslide and through the course of my healing, I kept hearing how I had been "initiated." The first time I heard this was from a shaman in the Arizona desert. The second time was in conversation with an esteemed Jungian psychologist. The number of times thereafter were in the countless books I read on healing from trauma and in courses with bestselling author and meditation teacher Joe Dispenza. So, what is trauma an initiation to?

Mystical schools of thought indicate that surviving trauma initiates one into a new reality. Initiation brings a deeper and greater awareness to feeling—to that we cannot see but can sense—to our interconnectedness as people and cultures and to life beyond the death of the body. It is the spiritual death of the old way of being and rebirth into an awakened and transformed life. Scientifically speaking, it has been shown via brain scans that the possibility exists for other parts of the brain to become lit up and more active in posttraumatic growth. This would indicate that new neural pathways are forming, and the brain is developing in different and novel ways.[11]

I felt that for me, it was an initiation to a deeper level of empathy than I had previous to the mudslide. I remember just weeks before the event driving along the beautiful Santa Barbara coast beneath the mountains while the deejay on the radio spoke of the flooding in Texas and people being displaced and losing their homes. Hearing that brought me sadness and sympathy and also a sense of awareness that I had no capacity for understanding what all of those people were experiencing. After the mudslide, just a few weeks later, my ability to relate to others who had experienced loss and suffering was more authentic and connected than it had been previously. I'm not saying that any person's experience, even in the same traumatic event, is alike or that we need to expose ourselves to all manner of traumas to understand and empathize with those who have been through them, but I'm just saying that such heightened and deepened compassion can result from surviving a traumatic experience. My conclusion is that surviving trauma is an initiation into a more interconnected, appreciative, and divine experience of life.

. . . .

EXERCISE: YOUR INITIATION

Although it can be a struggle in the wake of trauma to get past the realization that life is fleeting, can be snatched from us at any moment, and will include suffering, after you are on the other side of this epiphany, the temporal and expansive nature of life can become the focus. Do not beat yourself up if you are not there yet. Getting to this place of appreciation takes time, and it takes healing. Start exploring your initiation into this more complex and precious life by noticing and appreciating small things in your life. Initially, what you notice might be the beautiful color of a flower, the taste of a piece of fruit, a soft sweater, or the warmth of the sun. And then you can build upon the appreciation you felt for these things. How do you feel more connected to wonderful, loving people in your life, even if they were strangers who offered assistance or supplies? How do you appreciate life more? Are there things you realize you want to do that you've been putting off? Places to visit? How do you appreciate the world around you more? How do you appreciate your own strength more?

AN EXAMPLE OF REFRAMING: KATHY AND AMY ELDON'S STORY

Kathy Eldon is the mother of Amy Eldon and the late Dan Eldon. Kathy and Amy are radiant and dynamic, full of life and a desire to make life better for so many in the world. In the 1960s, Kathy, an American from Iowa, married a British exchange student named Mike Eldon and then moved to England, where she gave birth to Dan and then Amy. After several years, the family moved to Kenya.

Kathy and Mike taught their children the importance of service and help-ing those less fortunate. At the age of fourteen, Dan was raising money for a young Kenyan girl undergoing open-heart surgery. At the age of nineteen, he was organizing aid trips to Malawi refugee camps with friends and his then sixteen-year-old sister, Amy. Kathy encouraged him to draw, write, and photo-graph as a way to express his feelings. His journals, which feel reminiscent of Peter Beard, are stunning, capturing the essence of the wildness of life and what it means to be human. Hearing of the famine in Somalia, Dan immediately flew there to photograph the situation to share it with the world. The photo-graphs caught the eye of international news agency Reuters, who promptly hired Dan—the youngest photojournalist who had ever worked there. He was on assignment in Somalia on July 12, 1993, when an angry mob turned on him and three other journalists after the US Marines bombed a building thought to hold a warlord council. There were no warlords, and instead, many innocent civilians were murdered. Dan and the other journalists brought by survivors to photograph the scene were killed in the ensuing riot.

Having your son and your brother murdered by an angry mob is an unspeakable tragedy and trauma. Both Kathy and Amy could have caved in upon themselves and become bitter and withdrawn from the world. Instead, they channeled their grief, which Kathy says gave her "a tremendous amount of energy," and turned it into something to benefit and uplift other young activists around the world. They each went through intense periods of griev-ing: Kathy was unable to eat much of anything and crashed her car twice when she envisioned Somalia; Amy experienced panic attacks and struggled to process her grief while at college surrounded by carefree peers. Still, they explained that instead of letting that grief stay inside festering, they chan-neled the love they had for Dan into creative projects that went out into the world. They began writing books together, and their guided journal on loss and grief, *Angel Catcher*, continues to be a bestseller twenty years after they wrote it. They have hosted and produced television series, they have written seven books between the two of them, they fought for a film on Dan's life to be made called *The Journey Is the Destination*, they published Dan's journals, and they founded the Creative Visions Foundation in 1998 to support other activists to use their creativity to make the world a better place. During our interview, Amy told Kathy, "I don't know how you did it, Mom," to which Kathy replied, "There was no other choice." Amy considers her parents' fo-cus on transforming Dan's death, as a force for good rather than on revenge and retribution, a big factor in her own healing.

When I asked what had most helped them alchemize their grief and trauma of losing a loved one, it wasn't therapy or healers. "We were living in England. They don't really do therapy over there, or at least they didn't then," they said. They credit books they read as touchstones for wading through and transmuting their grief. *After Grief* by Hope Adelman and *Living in the Light* and *No Way Out but Through* by Shakti Gawain are the three titles that helped them most. Kathy explained that her own version of art therapy really helped her—she would draw her feelings, write, journal, listen to music, and dance. "Don't let those feelings clog you up. Don't keep them in; let them out, express them," Kathy urges. For both Kathy and Amy, creative expression has been paramount to their healing and their pivot toward living joyfully as well as creating a legacy for Dan that will live on forever. Kathy stresses that although some people might view her projects as grandiose, any sort of creative project—planting a garden, painting a mural—channeling the grief, and naming it for the person you have lost, will help. Kathy shares, "As I have discovered, the more imaginatively we delve into our sadness, the greater our capacity for joy will be when we eventually emerge from our tunnel of darkness. For humans are capable of rising above their sorrow to regenerate and expand. We can even learn to dance again—and one day, perhaps, even to fly."[12]

Forgiveness is another big piece of what helped them both move on. Kathy describes in her memoir *In the Heart of Life* her anger and resentment for the Somalis and feeling she would never be able to forgive them for killing Dan. In 1997, on the way to the United Nations for a screening of *Dying to Tell the Story*, a film they had produced on the dangers of photojournalism, their cab driver, Ebrahaim, was Somali. Kathy shared Dan's story and the fact that he had loved Somalis. Ebrahaim listened carefully, and when he stopped at a traffic light, turned and said, "Your son and the journalists should not have been killed. It was a terrible mistake. The people of Mogadishu are ashamed of what happened. On behalf of all Somalis, I ask your forgiveness." Kathy responded, "Thank you, Ebrahaim. I hate what the Somalis did, but I understand why they did it. I have forgiven the Somali people." Kathy shares that as soon as the words came out of her mouth, she knew they were true, and she was free from carrying the burden of blame and anger. She reiterates that forgiveness isn't actually for the transgressor, it is for you. It frees *you*.

Both Kathy and Amy emphasize the idea that through having known such all-encompassing sorrow, grief, and trauma, their joy becomes that much more visceral. The contrast of having sunk so low and knowing that dark place exists makes you appreciate beauty, love, and life that much more. In an article for a Boston University publication, Amy shared: "Over time, I found that pain visited less frequently, and when sorrow washed through me, it wasn't as deep or intense as it had once been. When I felt happy it was bliss because I had known the extremes of sadness. My worst nightmare had become a reality, and I survived— reborn through my grief, profoundly aware of how precious life really is."[13] Kathy and Amy's story is a great example of how reframing begins and evolves. In part 2 of this book, we'll dive into different healing modalities to help you on your way.

PART 2

Healing Modalities

There are many effective tools and therapies for dealing with trauma, and I've investigated every one that appeared on my radar! This is by no means a comprehensive list, but these are the modalities and people who most significantly helped me and the others I interviewed. Because I believe in a holistic approach, in which all facets of the self must be addressed for healing to be successful and lasting, I have broken down the modalities into the physical, emotional, and spiritual arenas.

It is important to trust your intuition and your feelings when embarking on a new therapy. I am not a doctor, and everything I offer here is just that, an offering of what worked for me or others I interviewed. If there is any question as to whether a therapy might be a good fit for you, consult with a doctor. For most people, there is a timeline on which healing takes place. One kind of therapy can be helpful if it's used at the right time but can be less so if applied too early in the healing process. Listen to yourself. As my sister, Lucy, and I have been saying for years on our Wild Precious Life Retreats, YOU are your own best guide. Healers and practitioners, and even authors immersed in this, are all here to help and support you on your path toward transformation. Yet only you can know what feels right and when. You are the one who ultimately heals you. Nobody does it for you or to you. We all have an innate and intrinsic ability to heal and evolve. Each practice, tool, book, and practitioner is just a suggestion, merely a torch to illuminate your way.

That being said, you need not be alone because we all need help. There is great value in having a witness to your own miraculous discoveries and healing triumphs. A partner, friend, healer, or therapist can act as a helpful and empowering mirror reflecting back your epiphanies, release, and strength. In my experience, these healing practices serve as a way to reconnect with our best versions of ourselves, our intuition, and our spirit. So, remember that if you try something that feels like *too much* or wrong, you can speak up and even end the session. It might not be right for you right now, or it might not be right for you ever.

This is critical to remember: If something doesn't work for you, it just wasn't the right therapy for you, and in no way does it indicate that you failed. That particular therapy just wasn't effective for you. Or it might have been the wrong practitioner or the wrong time. Trauma expert and psychologist Pat Ogden emphasizes the importance of interviewing several therapists before deciding to work with someone. There have to be connection, chemistry, trust, and safety because the therapist/client relationship is so intimate. So, if something isn't working, and you don't feel the potential, perhaps find another practitioner or simply explore another form of treatment. We are all individuals with nuanced and unique experiences, so there is no one-size-fits-all approach to healing. The last thing we want to feel in our healing journey is that we have failed. Ogden corrected me on this in our interview when I said that with movement therapies, I just want to get "it" out. She stopped me and said,

A lot of people think you can discharge the trauma by jumping around and moving. I don't hold with that. I think movement is a good thing, especially if you've gone toward immobilizing responses, but if you're using it to discharge energy, it's a temporary resource that can be very beneficial, but I wouldn't say it's part of my method. Implying that you have to get something *out* of your system can be confusing because when it comes back, you feel like you failed.

She emphasized that therapy is not about getting the trauma out but rather integrating all of our experiences and sensations, including our trauma.

Interestingly enough, when we have a particularly powerful healing session, we might feel a bit worse right afterward. Especially when we are healing energetically and emotionally, a lot can shift during a session that we can't necessarily put our finger on, but the movement of stagnant traumatic hooks can sometimes almost feel like a physical detox. I have had experiences where, after energy work, I felt a bit nauseated, tired, and I had a headache for a day or so afterward. This isn't a bad thing, and it doesn't mean that the therapy failed. In fact, quite the opposite: It can indicate that the therapy worked, and your body/mind/spirit is merely recalibrating as it expels the unhelpful energy and reorganizes without it. If you wind up feeling worse for more than a few days, it might mean another session or another therapy is a good idea to keep things moving and at a faster pace.

Another note about practitioners is that we are all works in progress, including therapists and healers. Although we can't expect anyone, including those helping us, to be perfect and have it all figured out, in my experience the treatment, whatever it might be, is more effective if there is trust, respect, and connection with the practitioner. Practitioners are human, and all of us have shortcomings and flaws. Resist the temptation to thrust a practitioner onto a pedestal or think that anyone knows you better than you.

In all healing modalities, if you distill them down, there is a through line of nature as a powerful healer. The link back to nature as healer is obvious in aromatherapy and flower essence work, but it exists even in a clinical practice such as eye movement desensitization reprocessing therapy (EMDR), which is successful because of the way it restores calmer, more balanced biological circuitry in the brain. In honoring the miracle of the human body and its autonomic processes for healing and growth, these modalities and tools move our egos and intellectual overthinking selves out of the way so that healing can unfold as it naturally does in animals, plants, ecosystems, and humans.

In the second half of this book, I'll provide a short explanation of what each therapy is and how it works and then share the way the participant experienced it, both during and afterward. I also include ideas for what you might do at home on your own, if that is a possibility. Resources for finding a practitioner within your area and budget are also listed. Again, if cost is an issue, don't be afraid to ask about sliding scales or pro bono sessions. Finally, I'll outline what treatments are best for certain types of trauma and if any symptoms or situations would make them a poor fit. Please keep in mind that these guidelines are not exhaustive.

I encourage you to consult with a doctor before embarking on any treatment plan. Each person is unique in their physiology and circumstances, and just because something worked at a certain pace or in an effective way for me does not ensure that you will have the same result or that it is a safe and appropriate therapy for you to try.

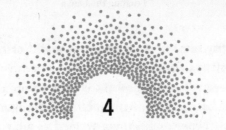

4

Move It!

Movement Therapies

Trauma interferes with the brain circuits that involve focusing,
flexibility, and being able to stay in emotional control. A constant
sense of danger and helplessness promotes the continuous secretion
of stress hormones, which wreaks havoc with the immune system
and the functioning of the body's organs. Only making it safe for
trauma victims to inhabit their bodies, and to tolerate feeling what
they feel, and knowing what they know, can lead to lasting healing.

BESSEL VAN DER KOLK, *THE BODY KEEPS THE SCORE*

Throughout my family's evacuation from the mudslide, losing our house, and then through my recovery, I came to deeply understand that my true physical "home" is my body. Tending to it and keeping it clear, healthy, and happy is critical to moving past a traumatic experience and living a dynamic life.

When we are traumatized, our bodies have a visceral autonomic response. Our brains and bloodstream are flooded with cortisol and adrenaline, and blood is shunted away from organs such as the stomach, intestines, brain, and liver to make more energy available for running and/or fighting. After the traumatic event is over and the threat has passed, all of this energy must be discharged and released so that the body can recalibrate and harmonize. If this doesn't happen, fear is stored in the tissues, affecting the overall ecosystem of the body. Consider the Japanese method of *ikejime*, in which fishers humanely kill fish so that they do not experience stress and fear. Fish killed by this method are sought after for their superior taste because of the absence of the unsavory flavors stress and fear leave behind. Not that we are going to be making a meal of ourselves!

The experiences of heart transplant recipients help us understand how profoundly memories and traumas can be stored in human tissues and organs. In his book *Becoming Supernatural,* Joe Dispenza, bestselling author, researcher, and international speaker, shares the story of Claire Sylvia, a forty-seven-year-old professional dancer who had a strong desire for fast food and Snickers bars after her heart transplant. These foods were some of her eighteen-year-old heart donor's favorites before his death in a motorcycle accident. Even more compelling was a trial that resulted from a heart transplant recipient having vivid dreams about being murdered. Her detailed physical description of the perpetrator, his clothing, the weapon, and the time and place of the crime led to his identification, arrest, and conviction for the rape and murder of her heart donor. She had never met her donor and did not know anything about the murder, and yet the memory of it was stored in the tissues of her transplanted heart!

Understanding the physiological effects of trauma is a powerful motivator to move! Recognizing the direct physical impact that thoughts and emotions have on our bodies is profound. Working *with* the body's innate healing capacity to release old traumatic sensations and emotions and restore the body to its natural state of homeostasis, balance, and harmony is like returning to a safe, nurturing home. Our bodies are our homes for this lifetime. Let us work with them, honor them, and keep them clear of traumatic residue.

In clearing residues of stress and fear from in our organs and tissues, we restore our nervous system and optimize bodily functions with efficient circulation of blood and lymph. This is why therapies that involve moving and/or manipulating the physical body must be part of the overall healing process after trauma. These therapies become a gateway to what lies beyond and underneath.

Norma Bastidas found that intense exercise was a way to reacquaint herself with her body, discharge pain from her past, and continue her healing. She was born in Mazatlán, Mexico, one of five children, and she endured rape and sexual abuse by her grandfather and uncle after her alcoholic father died when she was eleven years old. At the age of nineteen, and desperate to escape Mexico, she was offered a modeling job in Japan. The "job" turned out to be a cover for a sex trafficking operation, and she was stripped of her passport, held prisoner, and sold to the highest bidder in Japan. She eventually escaped and made her way to Canada, where she married and had two sons. Following her divorce, her eldest son was diagnosed with a genetic blindness disorder. She channeled her grief, anger, depression, and adrenaline into running. She says she started running "because I couldn't breathe." She needed a healthy outlet after bouts with eating disorders and substance abuse.

Bastidas went on to win the world record for longest triathlon as a woman in 2012. She swam, biked, and ran a route often used by sex traffickers from Cancún, Mexico, to Washington, DC, covering 3,762 miles. Using the publicity, she seized the moment to talk about what had happened to her and raise awareness about sex trafficking. "I had to do a world record to earn the right to say what happened to me," she shared with me. In an earlier interview with CNN, she said, "I cannot undo what has been done. But by living large, I'm empowering every single victim. Somebody who was once living a nightmare is now living out her dreams. Because that is what a world record is, it's a dream."

Developing a healthy and loving relationship with herself and her body was and continues to be a critical piece of Bastidas's healing. "Running for me is the closest thing I have to experiencing love at first sight, reclaiming my body after punishing it for so long with eating disorders and bad relationships. Running was like a celebration of my body, it felt good. I need to pursue things that bring me more joy."

SHAKING THERAPY/TRE

Shaking is a natural response of the body to discharge fear. As trauma therapist Peter Levine writes in his book *Waking the Tiger*, animals in the wild do not experience posttraumatic stress disorder (PTSD) in part because they shake to release the tension from their bodies as soon as they are out of danger. Full-body trembling is a way of regulating different states of nervous system activation, ultimately allowing the animal to move easily from one state to the other and back again.

Human beings, on the other hand, often hold on to fight-or-flight sensations that arise during trauma; then the fear and stress are stored in the body. If the heightened arousal state related to the trauma is not addressed, healed, and released, it can become a person's resting set point. The body makes this heightened state of arousal a "new normal," which has negative short- and long-term effects on the body's hormonal, immune, metabolic, and cardiovascular functions.

David Berceli, an international expert on trauma intervention who has spent decades studying and working to heal traumatized people in countries such as Uganda, Palestine, and Lebanon, developed a modality referred to as trauma releasing exercises (TRE). The series of exercises causes the natural reflex of shaking to occur, which triggers relaxation of the muscles. When the body relaxes and tension is released, the brain produces new hormones that aid in healing.

Berceli's exercises are designed to help release the psoas muscle, which connects the lower spine to the pelvis. The psoas has been called the muscle of the soul; in her book *The Power Source,* Lauren Roxburgh writes that Taoists believe it connects us to our ancestry as well as to our intuition. In Chinese medicine, there are acupressure points about four fingers' width to the side of the belly button, on both sides, where the psoas can be gently massaged while a patient is lying down. These points, referred to as the *heavenly pivot,* are where we "pivot" when a traumatic event happens. Through processing and healing the traumatic event we turn in the direction we and our lives need to go, ultimately toward the divine, practitioners and patients believe. Interestingly, the psoas receives its nerve signals from an acupuncture point over the spine (the psoas originates on the spine and wraps around to the front of the body, connecting to the pelvis) called the *gate of destiny.* The gate of destiny point holds and sends a great deal of power through the psoas to the heavenly pivot point, supporting and energizing the redirection of our lives after trauma toward the fulfillment of one's destiny. When we are still processing the traumatic event, we can hold the energy in the psoas, making it tender and uncomfortable, and delay the expansion and growth to which we've been initiated. Releasing the psoas can lead to healthy trembling in the body that discharges negative emotions and allows us to move forward.

When we clear old feelings associated with past trauma, we are free to connect more with the present moment and our intuition. Berceli's research has shown that vibrating the body either with a machine or through TRE exercises leads to faster healing, a reduction in pain, and relief from haunting emotions associated with trauma. Berceli's method has been used effectively with veterans and refugees worldwide.[1]

At the point in my own journey when I stumbled upon shaking as a means for moving through my own PTSD, I was feeling frustrated that I wasn't "further along." Panic attacks were haunting me, and although I had done so much work in terms of processing and healing, I still felt the aftershocks of dark thoughts and hypervigilance. A friend reminded me of our wise, kind, and direct prenatal yoga teacher, who had helped my friend through the dark moments of her marriage falling apart and postpartum depression. I had been in her prenatal class right after the mudslide, so she knew my story.

I scheduled a time to meet with her alone, anticipating some yoga moves and mudras (symbolic hand gestures) for trauma release and healing. After she caught up on where I was, on all levels, she had me move to the floor and showed me not a series of yoga postures but a series of strange-looking shaking exercises: one standing pigeon-toed with my knees bent; another lying on my back with all my limbs shaking. (Now I recognize that both these exercises are meant, in part, to release the psoas.) She instructed me to move through these exercises "like an earthquake" daily for at least fifteen minutes.

The lymphatic system, responsible for removing waste and toxins from the body while also circulating infection-fighting white blood cells, is the only system in our bodies without a pump. That means we must manually move the lymph in our bodies through breath, movement, massage, and—you guessed it—shaking! During a traumatic event, the lymphatic system slows down, so it is even more important to activate it during the healing and recovery process.

I must say, the specificity of these shaking exercises made them feel like a bit of a chore. My overactive thinking brain was trying so hard to do them "correctly" that my actual release felt limited. Still, it provided an introduction to the idea and practice of shaking to help my body, mind, and spirit.

During the Covid-19 lockdown in spring 2020, I rediscovered an old favorite teacher, Taryn Toomey, and a new one, Julianne Hough. Toomey's online studio, The Class, was a perfect outlet for me. Her routines incorporate jumping and shaking the body to release old, stored energy. The realization of how much calmer and at peace I felt after her classes was such a gift and crystallized for me how effective this strategy is for clearing stuck energy and the aftereffects of trauma. This was also true for Bastidas: Through physical exertion, she was able to compost some of her trauma.

Another example of healing through movement is Hough's story. Dance was a career, "a way to express myself, feel successful, and earn money," says Hough, who was discovered for her talent and became famous for it on *Dancing with the Stars*. But dance, for her, was much more than that. In looking back, she realizes that dance was always her safe place and a form of healing and therapy from childhood trauma. It was a way to voice and express through her body when she wasn't able to speak for herself: "If I hadn't had that outlet of movement, of dance, of expression, I think I would have had much more limiting beliefs, and that would have changed the trajectory of my life." Dance gave her a way to release and alchemize some of the trauma from childhood.

Hough became passionate about researching biology, chemistry, and energetics by studying qigong, tai chi, ecstatic dance, kundalini yoga, and other modalities to begin to formulate a program to help herself and others release trauma and stagnant energy and "wake up and feel alive." The result is Kinrgy, an online studio she first unveiled in person on tours with Oprah Winfrey and Tony Robbins.

Kinrgy incorporates three key elements: movement, breath, and visualization. There is intention in the order of the guided exercises. Each session begins by helping to unlock and open a channel of release in the body. Following release, the space created by discharging old stagnation is invited to fill with the feminine energy we all have, including men. Hough shares that this is a critical step in healing issues in the part of her body known as the sacral chakra. Lingering shame from sexual abuse and endometriosis had manifested in this part of her body. Often emotions can manifest into physical symptoms if they aren't permitted an outlet of expression.

Moving that energy up and out through visualization opens up the possibility of surrendering to the divine feminine inside and outside ourselves. By connecting to the feminine energy of the earth, which is also thought of as the mother, we allow ourselves to be held and nurtured. There is space for us to fall apart and then lovingly put ourselves back together in a way in which we are more empowered, free, and alive. It is challenging to surrender to this feminine energy because our society celebrates being tough rather than the alternative of releasing and letting go. Ultimately, surrendering and letting it go is much better for us emotionally as well as physically.

Kinrgy offers a way to reclaim our power, our sensuality, and our bodies. It gives people a platform to move their bodies, feel their bodies, and experience the ecstasy of being free energetically and sensually. Most women, especially those who have experienced sexual abuse, are familiar with the feeling of being unsafe or uncomfortable because of our sexuality. Often, we can become dissociated from our bodies and their sensations as a result of sexual abuse. Hough offers a way to reconnect with and celebrate our bodies and our sensuality. She says,

> Pleasure is not supposed to be a reward; pleasure is a state of living
> a full life. We've been taught to think that we need someone else
> to wake that up for us. But that ecstatic state is within us; we don't

need anybody to gift that to us because it's already inside of us. And then it's your choice if you want to share that with someone else. But it's not that someone needs to give that to you or wake you up. The prince is not coming to free you from your tower. You get to create whatever you want within your tower and outside of it.

. . . .

FOR YOU:

Many movement classes are offered online. Some to check out are Kinrgy, Dance Church, Taryn Toomey's online studio, 305 Fitness, and Ailey Extension. Roxburgh also offers trampoline and jumping sequences on her website laurenroxburgh.com.

If you're more of a do-it-yourselfer or don't have the budget, simply commit to ten to twenty minutes a day to jump, bounce on a rebounder (a mini trampoline), dance, or otherwise shake your body. It can be as simple as turning on some favorite tunes and letting go!

Three Moves for You

1. Turn on some of your favorite upbeat music and start by gently shaking your body. This might turn into dancing around the room!

2. Transition from dance into jumping jacks for the length of one song. You can break up the jumping jacks with freestyle dance if you are so moved: twelve jumping jacks and then twelve beats of dancing, and so on.

3. Ground your feet, and gently swing your outstretched arms from side to side twelve times. Let your whole torso and your head and neck follow your arms. I often feel (and hear!) my spine and neck release with this move.

Your body, brain, and spirit will thank you, and you will begin to notice shifts in your life. It is also important to note that although vigorous movement can temporarily release and discharge energies, emotions, and anxieties, as trauma expert Ogden points out, this is a temporary shift. She emphasizes this so that when the undesirable feelings, thoughts, or symptoms return, we don't feel like we have failed at "getting something out of the body." The goal of trauma therapy, Ogden explains, is to integrate parts that hold the trauma in the body, integrate parts of you that judge your reaction to the trauma, and integrate and recalibrate the nervous system. Parts of us can be shut down or splintered off during and following a trauma, particularly physically, because we may physically have been unable to move or may have endured painful or unwanted physical sensations. Reconnecting to, reawakening, and recalling the parts of us that shut down or compartmentalized the trauma is essential to our healing and becoming whole. Ogden counsels that movements and body-centered practices such as deep breathing, self-touch, lengthening the spine, and dropping the shoulders are all ways to reconnect with your bodily sensations in a healthy way that feels good. That's why for me, an exercise practice is part of my daily self-care routine; it does make me feel better and help me stay healthy and strong, but it is not a one-time singular therapy.

David Berceli also offers his TRE sequences on his website, traumaprevention.com, along with resources for finding TRE certified trainers wherever you live.

Whole-body vibration platforms are another way to integrate shaking into your exercise routine. Gyms and physical therapy clinics often have them, and you can buy your own to use at home. Squatting, pushups, and other bodyweight exercises take on a new dimension of shaking with this kind of equipment, found to reduce back pain, increase strength, and even slow loss of bone mass with aging. Simply standing on the platform of one of these machines can help start you on your shaking journey.

Who is it right for? Wrong for?

Shaking therapy is good for everyone. Even if you have a physical disability that restricts your movement, you can use your hands to jostle the muscles of your thighs, for example. This is something midwives recommend to mothers for relaxation during childbirth. A skilled bodyworker can help create the release of shaking therapy even if you are unable to create it yourself. Vibration platforms are another option for folks with different abilities.

Shaking therapy is especially good for anyone whose fight-or-flight rush coincided with being trapped, unable to run or move. This was true for me and would also be true for assault survivors whose trauma involved being held against their will.

One thing to note is that sometimes martial arts programs or model mugging programs (where people are taught how to fight off a simulated attack) can be retriggering if done without therapeutic support additionally. This might not be the case, but it is something to be aware of; we are all unique individuals, and what is cathartic and healing for one person might be distressing and retriggering for another person.

YOGA

Yoga has become a mainstream form of exercise, but actually, people in the area now known as India cultivated it in order to relax their bodies before meditation. More than a good workout, yoga has a strong focus on breathing and mindfulness. This is shown to reduce the size of the amygdala, the part of the brain responsible for fear, which often becomes overactive following a traumatic event.[2]

Another benefit of yoga is reconnecting with your body. Sometimes following a traumatic event we can become disconnected from our bodily sensations, or our relationship with our body in general might become distorted. We might have dissociated in the midst of a physically painful or uncomfortable situation. This may have helped us survive the event, but after the fact, this dissociation can become unhelpful and even potentially harmful. Practicing the physical poses and combining them with breathwork helps to reconnect us with our bodies in a way in which we can appreciate their strength, flexibility, and power.

Yoga instructor Brianna Turpin suffered the loss of her first child only three weeks after his birth following a healthy and normal pregnancy. She shares how her background in yoga helped her heal:

When I reflect on my own trauma, I can't help but think that my decade of yoga practice helped prepare me for loss and for healing. I am a huge proponent of a daily meditation and yoga practice because it helps us process the past and be more present in the now. But what I didn't realize was how much the practice was preparing me for what was to come. I believe yoga helped teach me presence, compassion, and the ability to move through tough emotions rather than skirt around them. Reconnecting with yoga after trauma looked surprisingly different to me. My yoga practices were gentle and in shorter spurts. Sometimes it felt safe and comforting to have a space to be in my body. And sometimes it felt scary and vulnerable. Yoga is always about connecting us to our truest and most essential selves. After trauma it's no different; it's a continual touchstone and reminder of our inner light.

The root of the word *yoga* itself means "union," Turpin explains. So one goal or intention in beginning yoga after a traumatic event would be to reconnect to the body, becoming whole again or perhaps for the first time. Yoga can act like a bridge between the brain and the body, she explains. Turpin believes that in reconnecting to sensations in the body while moving and stretching, reconnecting with our breath (taking deep breaths instead of short breaths), and reconnecting to our emotions by having a quiet time and space to turn inward, we help to integrate the disparate parts of the whole self. During the practice of yoga, we can begin to mend the connection between our minds, hearts, and bodies.

Turpin reminds us that even if you've decided intellectually to relax and let go, the body might remain on edge, bracing for the worst. Yoga helps activate the parasympathetic nervous system (our rest-and-digest state), in effect allowing us to relax. Experiencing this routinely enables us to establish this relaxed feeling as a new normal. Accessing and staying in a more open and relaxed yogic state can lead to our ability to access that state more and more of the time. We remind ourselves of our natural state, and we can maintain it and access it more easily and frequently.

Turpin also emphasizes the correlation between staying present while practicing yoga and staying present in our daily lives while not practicing yoga. She says,

> Those who have experienced trauma can find themselves living in the past, reliving painful memories again and again. Establishing a practice that helps us focus on the present moment also helps give us autonomy for the future. And perhaps most importantly, we learn the practice of interoceptive awareness; in essence, we learn to survey the inner landscape of our body, mind, and emotions.

This practice involves receiving, sensing, and evaluating signals from the body. Noticing how the breath is moving, what your thoughts are, and how your physical and emotional body feel. The alchemy and aim of this are to reembody your resilience, and your whole self.

I began practicing yoga fresh out of college while living in Los Angeles. For decades I thought about yoga as strictly my physical workout, and it did help me look leaner, but it also helped me feel calmer and better in my own skin. In looking back, taking up yoga correlated with my first forays into the energetic realms and alternative styles of healing. Perhaps the yoga relaxed me enough to be open to these new healing avenues?

Following the mudslide, I kept up my yoga practice and found it an excellent way to uncover, release, and recover. It felt comforting to be around other people but also not have to talk. Some days it was hard to "stay with myself," whereas on other days epiphanies would come from the quiet depths I allowed myself to be still enough to access and listen to. It's sort of like those brilliant ideas and discoveries you have while in the shower or while driving, when you are in a relaxed state of allowing. Yoga gives me time and space to allow and to receive *myself.* As Turpin has mentioned, it has granted me another way in which to access, see, and embrace my whole self.

FOR YOU:

Yoga has become extremely popular, and there are studios popping up all over the place. There are also some excellent free yoga classes online! CorePower Yoga (corepowerondemand.com) offers a collection of free classes for intermediate to advanced yogis, and Yoga with Adriene is an approachable YouTube channel for those of you just getting started or wanting a gentler approach.

There is something to be said for practicing in person and with a community, but the convenience of taking an online class on your own time in your own space has been a gift to me during the Covid lockdown and thereafter. Yoga Works (yogaworks.com) is where I first learned yoga in Santa Monica. They have moved all of their classes online, and they offer high-quality, well-trained instructors.

Yoga is a bit like therapy in that all instructors and classes have their own personality and style. Take a few classes with a few different teachers to find one that resonates with you.

I love a spiritual vinyasa class that incorporates music. Vinyasa is a more active yoga style that gets my heart rate up, which helps me move and access emotions and endorphins more easily. There is always the option to slow down and take a child's pose (a resting pose) in any class. I love Turpin's classes, which can be found at briannayoga.com. Shiva Rea, a teacher whose classes I frequented years ago, incorporates a lot of energy and spirit into her classes. She offers classes at shivarea.com.

A Beginning Yoga Series

1. Stand up straight, with your feet hip distance apart and your hands at your sides. Inhale deeply, feeling and hearing the breath fill your body. Exhale, and imagine the breath traveling down the length of your body and out the soles of your feet. Feel yourself rooted and connected to the earth.

2. Inhale again, this time raising your arms up above your head. As you exhale, bend at the waist and touch your toes or your shins, depending on your flexibility. Keep a slight bend in your knees if that feels better.

3. Inhale and lift your upper body halfway with a straight spine, hands on shins and upper and lower body perpendicular to one another.

4. Exhale and gently fold over your legs again.

5. Inhale and rise all the way up with a flat back and reach your arms above your head.

6. Exhale and bring your arms to prayer position in front of your heart or down by your sides.

7. You can repeat this several times.

Who is it right for? Wrong for?

Really, anyone can benefit from yoga. Even if you have an injury or disability, there are classes and teachers who can help tailor things for you so that you can still reap the benefits of a yoga practice. If you're someone who suffers from dissociative patterns, speak with your doctor before exploring movement therapies.

If you are new to yoga, start with a beginner class or one geared toward relaxation and restoration. Always listen to your body, and if something doesn't feel right, particularly in a joint or your lower back, back out of the pose. There is a difference between strengthening and straining.

I've had people express that they can't stand yoga because they need more aerobic activity, and they get bored. Again, there are so many different styles of yoga classes and teacher personalities! If you tend to get bored and need a little more action, opt for a vinyasa class with music. If vinyasa classes with music are too fast and too loud for you, try a more mellow flow class or an ashtanga or Iyengar style class. Ashtanga style classes traditionally consist of the same sequence of poses performed in order. Iyengar yoga focuses on precision and holding poses for a length of time. I also love a good kundalini yoga class. Kundalini yoga is meant to activate the energy held in the base of our spines and channel it upward, in a spiral, activating all of our chakras. It is a good blend of physical and spiritual.

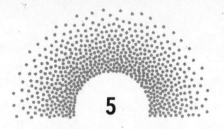

5

Nature!

How to Heal Yourself with Scents, Flowers, and Plants

Another portal into our inner worlds can be accessed through plants and flowers. Indigenous civilizations and medicine men and women have been using plants and flowers for their healing properties since the beginning of recorded time. In our Western culture, where we expect even alternative remedies to be supported by scientific testing, the superpowers of plants and flowers have been largely dismissed. Scientific studies are enormously expensive, and no one stands to earn back that cost as a purveyor of plant remedies. This helps to explain why there are not more studies conducted in these natural areas.

When first exploring the potential of these remedies, I felt more curiosity than confidence in their healing potential. I am happy to say that they've surpassed my expectations.

AROMATHERAPY

Aromatherapy, the therapeutic use of essential oils, is a centuries-old practice and has been a personal passion of mine my whole life. The potency and healing power of oils derive, at least in part, from a scientifically recognized impact of scents on the emotional centers of the brain.

While I sat trapped, terrified, and shivering on my bathroom counter in the darkness and cold of the night of the mudslide, a bottle of rose-scented soap just happened to be near enough for me to grab. I used it to wash my hands with the little bit of water left in the pipes. That rose scent gave me a sense of sweetness and supported me in believing that my family and I would be okay. An even greater gift was that a bottle of an essential oil blend, Inner Peace, by Lotuswei, was also on the counter with me. After I'd washed my hands and regained some sort of mental clarity, I pumped some Inner Peace into my hands and inhaled deeply. I invited myself to meditate and to allow the calming effects of the oils to bring my brain and body to a place where I could not only endure being trapped but also could potentially think clearly enough to find my way out.

A review study published in the *Journal of Neuroscience* details the connection between the olfactory nerves, which process smell, and other parts of the brain that process our emotions:

> The olfactory sense has a unique intimacy with emotion. Unlike other senses, olfactory neuroanatomy is intertwined, via extensive reciprocal axonal connections, with primary emotion areas including the amygdala, hippocampus, and orbitofrontal cortex (OFC). Olfactory stimulation can directly activate amygdala neurons, bypassing the primary olfactory cortex, before arriving at the secondary (association) olfactory cortex situated in the middle of the OFC.[1]

Put more simply, aromas have a direct impact on the parts of the brain responsible for our fight-or-flight emotions, which originate in the amygdala, and for the enduring activation that can ensue after a traumatic event. Medicinal properties of these oils can also be absorbed through skin. Some research has shown benefits for anxiety, depression, insomnia, and nausea as well.[2]

In the years since the mudslide, I have used essential oils throughout the day, every day. In the morning, I mist myself with a cedar oil for its grounding properties; then, depending on how I'm feeling, I'll also choose a blend for love, for protection, or for peace; sometimes I'll use all of them! And I always finish with The First, a fragrance I created with my sister, Lucy, as a way to bottle the essence of our Wild Precious Life Retreats.

For those who attend our retreats, the scent acts as an anchor to the feeling of expansiveness and peace they experienced on the retreat. For those unable to join us in person, we wanted the perfume to act as a portal to a sense of harmony and freedom. We honestly call it "a retreat in a bottle." Each essential oil in the perfume has its own properties: Juniper is detoxifying, honeysuckle is uplifting, rose geranium calms fears, lavender is relaxing, sandalwood is grounding, and kumquat is energizing.

I use scents throughout the day. I keep them in my purse and in my car. Before bed, I apply some Inner Peace and sometimes lavender as well. After the mudslide, I began applying some magnolia oil on my inner wrist before bed because it has properties that help to ease posttraumatic states. I brought essential oils into the hospital with me when I gave birth to my two children to diffuse throughout the hospital room for their cleansing, purifying, and calming properties. I used them with greater intensity and deeper purpose during the Covid lockdown. In addition to the peace and protection they offered me, certain aromas could transport me to beautiful places around the world I was not physically able to visit.

FOR YOU:

Many essential oils are beneficial in healing from trauma and maintaining a balanced, happy, and healthy baseline. Following are some of my favorites and their properties. These oils can be combined or used one at a time. They can be diffused, applied topically (check to be sure they don't need to be diluted with a carrier oil like jojoba oil to avoid skin irritation), or ingested (again, check each oil to be sure this is safe). With certain oils, you can add a few drops to an eight-ounce glass of water and drink it or add them to your bath water for a good soak. I learned from healers well versed in Chinese medicine that when applying oils to the skin, there are acupressure points where they are more effective: Apply them to the soles of your feet, your inner wrist closer to the thumb side, and your solar plexus. The spot on your inner wrist, thumb side, about an inch away from your wrist crease, is known as acupuncture point Lung 7, which correlates with restoring the adrenal glands. As we've already discussed, the adrenals are in overdrive while we are in a traumatic or PTSD state, so everything we can do to support and calm them is helpful. It's also beneficial to rub a few drops between your palms, hold your open palms near your face, and breathe deeply.

- **Rose geranium** calms fears and worry.

- **Magnolia** has antinociceptive (pain-blocking) benefits that decrease sensitivity to stress triggers.

- **Ylang ylang** has a sultry aroma and contains an antidepressant and antianxiety compound called *linalool*. A 2018 study on linalool found that it decreases anxiety and acts as an antidepressant when introduced into the body via ylang ylang aromatherapy.[3] In *The Power Source*, Roxburgh recommends rubbing a few drops of ylang ylang from your belly button down to your pubic bone to activate and nurture several key acupressure points. These points directly affect our hormones, creativity, and sexuality.

- **Frankincense** has been regarded as precious since biblical times, when it was used as currency. For centuries, monks have used it to enhance meditative states. It has properties that aid in stress relief, dispel negative emotions, and promote sleep.

- **Vetiver** soothes the nervous system, reduces anxiety, and helps relieve insomnia. If velvet were a smell, it would be the scent of this woody scented oil.

- **Neroli** has antidepressant and self-esteem-boosting properties and helps alleviate feelings of panic.

- **Cistus** (rock rose) was used in ancient Greece for its wound-healing abilities and as a beauty product because of its high polyphenol content. It is also widely used as an antiviral. It is a good oil to use to alleviate shock and soothe the heart, especially when feeling numb.

- **Eucalyptus and peppermint** both help with expansion and clearing of the lungs, thought to be one of the main places in our body where we hold grief.

- **Spikenard** is a woody smelling root with calming and grounding effects. Spikenard will help with mental hyperactivity of all kinds. It can help reduce emotional reactivity and intense emotions as well as aid sleep.

- **Helichrysum,** a flower that smells sweet and amber-like, is harmonizing and nurturing.

- **Sandalwood** grounds and calms the spirit and can also increase sensuality.

- **Lavender** is a popular scent for the promotion of relaxation, calm, and harmony.

Snow Lotus, Mountain Rose, Young Living, and DoTerra all offer high-quality oils easily accessed online. I also like Lotuswei oils. Lotuswei has an interesting and compelling philosophy, marrying essential oils and flower essences.

If you shop for oils in stores like Whole Foods, they will usually have testers you can smell to see what suits you. I would identify a few scents that speak to you both from an aroma standpoint and in terms of what healing support they can offer. Incorporate them into your daily routines. Create a ritual around their application to reap all the benefits.

Who is this right for? Wrong for?
If you are sensitive to certain aromas or have sensitive skin, check with your doctor, but most everyone can benefit from aromatherapy. Even those with anosmia (lack of smell) have been shown to benefit.[4]

FLOWER ESSENCES
Flower Power! For real. I thought there was no way flower essences could be a viable and effective therapy, and I was wrong. Edward Bach, a physician and homeopath, began experimenting and noting the effectiveness of different flowering plants and trees in the 1930s. He left his medical practice following World War I and moved to the English countryside, where he formulated thirty-eight flower essences, known as the Bach Original Flower Remedies. They are widely available. Each essence is derived from a different flower, plant, or tree and corresponds to an emotion. For example, aspen,

derived from the aspen tree, helps to calm fear and worry and brings a sense of security, which can be disrupted during a trauma.

Katie Hess is one of the most passionate and knowledgeable individuals making flower remedies available to the masses. She is a flower alchemist, author of *Flowerevolution,* and founder of Lotuswei, one of the world's leading floral apothecaries. With her signature elixirs featured in *O* (Oprah Winfrey's magazine), the *New York Times*, and the *Los Angeles Times*, her flower-powered community is thriving in more than fifteen countries. When I asked her to demystify the wonderfully magical and mystical world of flower remedies by stating how they actually work, she responded, "I think of it as floral Wi-Fi. People say that's so hard to believe because I can't see it with my eyes, but all it takes is a reflection on how our cell phones work, that we can send music and videos and photos across invisible waves that travel through space. Nobody questions it, we just use it."

Flower remedies work the same way: The energy of the flower is transmitted to our bodies. Hess explains that because flowers are the reproductive organs of the plant, they contain the most amount of the energy from the plant. Because every living thing emits its own unique energy, each plant and flower has its individual benefits for us. When distilled in water, the information and properties of the flower are stored in the water. When that water containing the flower essences joins with the water of your own body, the energy and benefits of the flower are transmitted. The flower remedies then flow to the meridian points in the body (the same points used in acupuncture) to release any stagnation and ultimately return us to our natural harmonious state. She emphasizes that flower essences are effective in helping to amplify the messages that belong to us and turn down the volume on the stories that don't belong to us. We store up to six to eight generations in our family lineage of information and patterning, patterns of thinking and feeling, good, bad, ugly, positive, wonderful, and limiting. The flower essences will ultimately go after what does not belong to us and show it to us so we can make a change or just simply turn the volume down so we can hear ourselves rather than a story that doesn't belong to us. This includes turning the volume down on the collective consciousness as well.

Hess observed that during 2020, a time of increased fear, anxiety, and anger globally, people regularly taking flower essences were immune to the collective consciousness. As a result, they were able to tap into their own inner wisdom and emotions rather than being at the mercy of the negative emotions in the collective.

Certain flower essences are especially good at alleviating symptoms of residual trauma. Hess says bee balm and spotted bee balm are unsurpassed at liberating unwanted symptoms that can linger following a traumatic event. Bee balm is particularly effective in healing past, older traumas and can be found in her Lotuswei blend Boundless Wisdom. Boundless Wisdom helps uproot unwanted sensations/feelings/reactions associated with a traumatic experience. Hess advises that a healing crisis can occur at the start of taking the remedy, followed by an intensification of the symptoms for about three to five days, and then they completely go away. This precipitated a little fear and resistance on my part because we're working on feeling better, not worse! Hess encouraged me that the remedy is never going to give us what we can't handle. Essentially, the remedies can make issues so apparent that you can't ignore them, motivating you to get angry or upset enough to address them, heal them, and release them. So don't chuck your bottle if things feel a bit more intense for the first few days to a week after you begin a remedy. Remember, it is better to release than to hold this detritus clogging your system.

For acute stress and simply feeling grounded and more at ease, Inner Peace is a milder blend that will not stimulate a healing crisis. Hess refers to Inner Peace as a "stabilizing" blend, whereas Boundless Wisdom goes deeper. The third blend she recommends in the most powerful and effective trifecta for healing trauma is called Luscious Embodiment. Luscious Embodiment contains squash blossom, her most effective remedy for sexual abuse. It also really helps with establishing healthy boundaries for yourself. She recommends working with all three of these essences for complete and thorough healing. You can take them either in the mist form, which you spray on yourself, or in the elixir form, which you put in your coffee, tea, or water and ingest. Take them five times a day or more during an acutely stressful or retriggering time. Follow your intuition on taking them one at a time for a few weeks before moving on to the next.

After reaching for that bottle of Inner Peace on the bathroom counter while trapped those five hours, I have continued to use it when I need a little help settling. It elicits calm and peace even under the most stressful circumstances.

Hess was correct in that I did have a bit of a healing "crisis" the first few days I took the Boundless Wisdom. I felt a bit more agitated and anxious in a generalized way. I upped my meditative practices and had outlets and people with whom to process my experiences and what was coming up for me to clear. I also determined that I am extremely sensitive to the remedies, so I didn't need quite as much as I was administering to myself, about five drops five times a day. When I backed off and also made it through those first few days, I did feel something had been lifted.

∙∙

FOR YOU:

Alexis Smart is a healer who splits her time between the Hollywood hills and the hills of the Greek islands, where she furthers her study of flower essences. Her ethereal looks, soft-spoken nature, and palatable empathy gave me hope that this might work. Back in my thirties I was a struggling actor disillusioned by the world of film and television. I suffered from self-doubt and anxiety, knowing I needed to make a life change but not knowing how or to what. Smart's quiet calm and wisdom allowed for me to feel seen and heard. Ultimately, the remedy she prescribed helped me. After the mudslide, I reached out again, and the trauma remedy she sent me helped with sleep and feelings of restlessness and fear.

Smart offers personal consultations and custom blends. She also offers a variety of preformulated remedies that she sells directly from her website with detailed instructions for how to take them, for how long, and so forth. She recommends Unburden, I Will, and Safe and Sound, in particular, for transforming the residue of trauma.

Lotuswei offers the blends I use and many others for different needs and outcomes. I also love the heart-opening series of flower essences: Infinite Love, Fierce Compassion, and Open Heart for healing relationships, self-love, and attracting and having more love in your life.

You could also create your own blend! For example, aspen is excellent for soothing anxiety and creating inner peace, rock rose helps neutralize panic by bringing forth more courage, and star of Bethlehem addresses the grief associated with trauma. Bach Original Flower Remedies are sold through Amazon and other online retailers.

Who is it right for? Wrong for?
Flower essences are not to be confused with essential oils and aromatherapy because they are scentless and are ingested, taken in drops under the tongue or in coffee, tea, or water. The Lotuswei line offers flower remedies in both the elixir form to be ingested and in mists (that smell wonderful) if you prefer that application. They are safe for

people of all ages, including children and pregnant women. They are gentle and effective and would be a good remedy at any time after trauma, particularly at the beginning.

NATURAL PROGESTERONE CREAM

In my pursuit of answers for healing trauma, I was led to a podcast interview by Dave Asprey of Bulletproof Coffee on adrenaline as it affects your overall health. Given what we know about how cortisol and adrenaline levels surge during a trauma and often remain elevated afterward (PTSD), my interest was piqued. Asprey's interview with Michael Platt, a former board-certified internal medicine doctor with nearly forty years of experience, was captivating and exciting. Platt, whose Platt Wellness Center is based in Rancho Mirage, California, has devoted his life to the study of the roots of illness and disease and traces many symptoms and diseases back to elevated adrenaline levels. He has published two books, *The Miracle of Bio-Identical Hormones*, which has been a bestselling health book in Germany for years, and *Adrenaline Dominance*. When I interviewed Platt for this book, he explained that the medical board became alarmed by his success rate of getting patients safely and effectively off of prescription drugs and attacked him for five years, costing him hundreds of thousands of dollars in his defense. Eventually he voluntarily surrendered his medical license in 2009. Platt expresses frustration and concern over the lack of education most doctors receive in hormones and how our medical system is significantly flawed by its close ties with the pharmaceutical companies. Considering research conducted by Danish physician and medical researcher Peter C. Gotzche, prescription drugs are the third leading cause of death after heart disease and cancer. Platt, in his straightforward approach to addressing hormone balance and management of insulin and glucose levels to prevent adrenaline spikes, asserts that fibromyalgia, irritable bowel syndrome, depression, attention deficit/hyperactivity disorder (ADHD), weight gain, addictions, colic in babies, bipolar depression, and PTSD can all be remedied simply by the application of bioidentical progesterone cream to the skin.[5] Again, consult with your doctor before using progesterone cream.

Progesterone is a hormone made primarily in the ovaries of women during their fertile years, but it is also made by the adrenal glands of men to produce testosterone and make sperm. Progesterone's job (in concert with another female hormone, estrogen) is to prepare the uterus to receive a fertilized egg. Along with its crucial role in making new life possible, progesterone has a potent impact on mood and sense of well-being. Its calming, soothing, mellowness-inducing effects are a main reason the discomforts of pregnancy are tolerable. Elevated levels of progesterone during ovulation are known to induce calm and increase libido while reducing anxiety; conversely, when progesterone levels drop just before menstruation, we get the phenomenon widely known as premenstrual syndrome (PMS). As progesterone levels tank postpartum, "baby blues," or postpartum depression, can result. Mood changes and insomnia before and during menopause are also linked to ebbing progesterone production.

Studying the calming effects of progesterone made a lightbulb go off for me personally. If you remember, I was pregnant when the mudslide hit, meaning my progesterone levels were significantly higher than they would have been otherwise. Furthermore, because I breastfed for nine months, even though progesterone levels drop off after birth, I was buoyed by prolactin, a hormone responsible for helping produce breast milk, which also secretes dopamine, providing feelings of happiness and euphoria. My lightbulb going off is linked to the fact that I didn't have a panic attack until *after* I was finished breastfeeding, for me indicating a link between my hormones and feelings of anxiety, fear, and distress. The natural progesterone and prolactin coursing through my body had helped me maintain a calmer, less adrenalized state.

During a trauma, adrenaline is released to provide fuel for the brain. This is helpful during the trauma, but overactive adrenaline following a trauma deteriorates our health and mood. Some signs that you have elevated adrenaline levels are getting up to pee in the middle of the night (glucose drops off at around 2:30 a.m., causing you to wake), cold hands and feet, neck tension, and teeth grinding. In Platt's experience, PTSD responds wonderfully to lowering levels of adrenaline simply by the application of a 5 percent progesterone cream (or 50 mg/pump). He makes his own bioidentical progesterone cream, and there are others on the market; Whole Foods even sells one made from wild yams.

I know this because a few months before listening to Platt, per my gynecologist's suggestion, I had bought a progesterone cream made from wild yams from Whole Foods in order to "reboot" my uterus following the birth of my second baby. I'm still not entirely sure how the reboot went, but I can tell you that I felt AMAZING with just a small pump of this magical cream. It can make you sleepy, which is why I put it on just before bed. My experience initially was of sleeping more soundly, feeling more responsive instead of reactive, and in general, loving it. I had forgotten about this magical cream until listening to the podcast and dug it out again. Although I experienced some benefits, I was uneasy about tinkering with my hormones, so I limited the use of the cream to a few weeks and then no longer felt I needed it.

. . . .

FOR YOU:

Considering the revocation of Platt's medical license, I must offer this disclaimer acknowledging that you understand that progesterone therapy could be dangerous if handled improperly and that I am not liable for any personal injury arising from any misuse of any products discussed here. Now that that's out of the way, if you meet the criteria for adrenaline dominance and you get the go-ahead from your doctor or naturopath, the cream I tried is a lower dose than Platt's. There are many other bioidentical progesterone creams on the market, and the cream form is more easily absorbed into the bloodstream than a pill. For most creams, it is recommended to apply a dime-sized amount of cream to the inner thighs, bottoms of the feet, or insides of the arms. For premenopausal women, the recommendation is to use the cream for fourteen days before your period. For menopausal women, you are advised to use the cream for twenty-one days and then give the body a break for seven days. And then repeat. As I mentioned, the cream made me sleepy, so I only applied it before bedtime.

Foods can stimulate progesterone production as well. Eating a diet rich in cabbage, kale, beans, soybeans, broccoli, cauliflower, nuts, spinach, pumpkin, brussels sprouts, and whole grains can stimulate progesterone, and eating bananas, shellfish, and walnuts can naturally lower the amount of estrogen in the body. When estrogen is lowered, there is a higher proportional amount of progesterone in the body.

Who is this right for? Wrong for?

Unlike many of the other therapies I've shared, natural progesterone might not be safe for everyone. There are some exciting studies on the use of progesterone as a treatment for women with PTSD, such as the Society for Women's Health Research reporting that "progesterone may be another treatment modality for women with PTSD. As [stated earlier,] progesterone is a precursor of ALLO (allopregnanolone, a neurotransmitter that mediates the fear response)."

Reproductive hormones such as progesterone, estrogen, and testosterone are incredibly complex, and their overall balance in the body is as important as the level of any one individual hormone. Side effects or negative effects from incorrectly using progesterone are not life threatening but can mean it does you more harm than good. Your best bet is to work with a naturopathic or integrative medicine physician who can support you in hormone-level testing and in using natural progesterone on the right schedule and in the right amount.

It is possible to manage natural progesterone therapy for yourself; if you choose to do so, refer to one or more of the books by John Lee, a respected authority on this topic, or go to Virginia Hopkins's website, virginiahopkinstestkits.com, for up-to-date information and access to quality progesterone creams, hormone testing, and guidelines. Although most evidence presented by these doctors and advocates of natural progesterone cream suggest that it does not increase risk of breast cancer or other types of cancer—in fact, most evidence suggests that it protects against these diseases—there is enough uncertainty about this to merit some caution if you are at high risk for cancer or have already survived it. This does not mean you should avoid natural progesterone altogether, but you might want to take special care to consult with a physician who understands its use before trying it.

Some sources promote natural progesterone as a good bet for men, but at this point, I'm suggesting it only as an option for women.

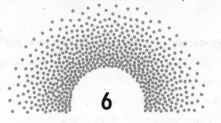

6

Chinese Medicine

C hinese medicine has been effective at alleviating physical and psychological symptoms for centuries.[1] Encompassing several branches covered here, acupuncture, gua sha, and qigong (energy cultivation), they can be explored one at a time and are most effective when combined and practiced as a holistic system.

ACUPUNCTURE

At the root of acupuncture and Chinese medicine in general is the belief that the natural state of all beings is one of balance. The philosophy is that heaven and earth merge in human beings, and when these two forces are harmonious, they manifest in healthy divine creation of all kinds. When we are out of balance, our body and soul crave to be brought back into alignment. Feeling out of balance is experienced uniquely by each person: One person might feel wired and have trouble sleeping, and another person might feel lethargic and not be able to get out of bed. We are distinctive individuals, and our symptoms manifest differently. Acupuncture is integrative medicine that aids in bringing a person back into balance by using tiny needles inserted into specific points in the body. It can be used to treat all manner of pain and illness, as well as psychological and emotional distress, by synching our human life force with the life force of nature. According to Johns Hopkins Medicine, "Acupuncture points are believed to stimulate the central nervous system. This, in turn, releases chemicals into the muscles, spinal cord, and brain. These biochemical changes may stimulate the body's natural healing abilities and promote physical and emotional well-being."[2]

Acupuncture was discovered thousands of years ago. Chinese medicine practitioner and qigong master Paul Fraser explains,

> Shamanic rituals designed to summon and harmonize the forces of heaven and earth within the body are described in the earliest discovered writings, some 7,000 years ago. These rituals amplified the forces of heaven and nature within the body, leading first to a discovery of qi, the animating force that permeates all of creation, including one's own body, and also the knowledge that each person's body contains all of the elements of the universe.

Following this discovery, practitioners were able to see that the forces of heaven and earth were contained in each person, along with the "gates" through which these forces entered and exited. These "gates" are known today as acupuncture points. If stagnation or symptoms manifested, balance could be restored through massage, stimulating the qi and blood flow and opening the gates through which the qi entered. As it became apparent that multiple gates needed simultaneous opening in order to restore harmony, the gates were wedged open by inserting needles just under the skin. First the needles were made of slivers of animal bone and jade, later from silver and gold (to attract either yin or yang forces), and today with stainless steel.

According to Minka Stevens, acupuncture moves things quickly and can immediately reset your nervous system. She also explains that in Chinese medicine, disease is thought of as an impediment to the body's natural state of flow. When symptoms arise, they are a manifestation of the stagnation and imbalance in the body. There may be many causes for the imbalance, from the simple to the severe. One may live in a harsh climate that adversely effects the body, eat and drink substances that aren't right for their bodies, have been traumatized, have genetic factors, or have been worn out though stress and overwork, just to name a few. Any state of imbalance can lead to all manner of symptoms physically, emotionally, and/or spiritually. These symptoms are a warning sign to let us know that in some way we are negating our own potential. The role of the acupuncturist is to identify where the blockage is and release it, thereby harmonizing the organs and systems in the body.

I have been receiving acupuncture for years and returned to Minka's table shortly after the mudslide. She had treated me for the usual host of issues: digestion, sleep, generalized anxiety, and prenatal care. Following the mudslide, she switched her approach with me to one called National Acupuncture Detoxification Association (NADA), often used on battlefields and for treating traumatic residue because of its focus on unwinding the sympathetic nervous system. As I discussed in chapter 2, when we are traumatized or facing a threat, our brains and bodies switch on the sympathetic nervous system, which elevates our heart rate and floods our system with adrenaline and cortisol in order to help us survive. Sometimes, we can get stuck in this sympathetic state instead of returning to the parasympathetic state of rest and relaxation. The NADA protocol helps our bodies let go of what we might have already worked through intellectually and emotionally by releasing neurotransmitters such as serotonin into the blood faster and more efficiently.

Kathleen Zisser is a Western medical doctor who practiced medicine affiliated with hospitals for years before leaving to start her own acupuncture clinic in Santa Barbara. She loves the holistic approach Chinese medicine emphasizes and the ability to spend more time with her patients. Zisser also relies on the NADA protocol to address trauma. She was part of a team deployed to administer this protocol to first responders right after the mudslide in Montecito. She explained that the sooner you can reach trauma and "deactivate the fear response," the better. The NADA protocol is an auricular one, meaning it is practiced on the ears. Needles are inserted into acupressure points in the ears, activating the vagus nerve, which is responsible for various internal organ functions such as digestion and heart and respiratory rate. This can also be achieved by putting ear seeds, tiny metal or ceramic balls, onto the points in the ears and leaving them there with small pieces of surgical tape. This allows for the points to stay activated and continue to help. You can even press on them for deeper release.

During the mudslide, my kidneys were also taxed by the excess adrenaline and cortisol released in a traumatic event. As Gianna de la Torre describes, in Chinese medicine the kidneys are seen as the "queen" of the body, ruling the yin, or feminine, energy, and the heart is seen as the "king" of the body, ruling the yang, or masculine, energy. When a traumatic incident occurs, Gianna says, the heart and the kidneys separate. "Trauma fragments us," she says. "We describe something as 'heart stopping,' literally because the heart energy recoils into its region, while the kidneys are all about fear, so they retreat into their region, creating imbalance with these major organs not communicating with each other." By unwinding this fear response in the body, we free up energy and communication between these two systems.[3]

Gianna is no stranger to this phenomenon. She was in the middle of acupuncture school and teaching yoga when her boyfriend was killed in a car accident. A tractor trailer in front of them broke loose from a truck and crashed through their windshield, killing her boyfriend while she was in the seat beside him. Although Gianna survived without much more than a few scratches on her physical body, inside she was shattered by grief and trauma and gripped by a fear of death and dying. She dropped out of school because she couldn't focus and had a depressed and doomed mindset about life, often thinking, "Why bother? What's the point?" For the first six months following his death, she didn't do any healing work. After that, something shifted, and she began her healing journey in earnest, focusing on acupuncture as a means to move all of that stagnant energy.

After my fear response had abated enough for my body to be receptive to further healing, Minka implemented a version of acupuncture called aggressive energy. This modality is used to release aggressive energies and elevated levels of stress in the body. Minka describes this approach as "a big reset for all of your organs, similar to rebooting your computer." This protocol draws on the belief that the five elements found in nature—water, fire, wood, earth, and metal—each correspond with a different organ. Kidneys are water, heart is fire, liver is wood, spleen is earth, and lungs are metal. The treatment is carried out by needling the most deeply tonifying points on the back, also known as shu points, which release tension and stagnation and are correlated with these organs. Minka was careful with me when she used this system because it can have a detoxifying effect, or healing reaction, which comes with letting go, but can make you fatigued and vulnerable for a day or two afterward.

Another protocol effective in treating trauma is called seven dragons. Dragons are thought of as messengers from heaven in Chinese medicine, analogous to angels in Western religions. Each of the seven dragon points can be needled in order to release and alchemize trauma. Paul Fraser outlines a detailed explanation for each of the dragon points:

The seven dragons:

1. Conception Vessel 15, "Dove Tail" (one point/dragon), the place where Qi bridges the diaphragm and enters the chest. The diaphragm is the merging of Yin and Yang forces in the body, where Heaven and Earth combine. This point acts as the lid to an alchemical vessel. It is the

influential point of the Pericardium, the muscle that contracts the heart, seen by the Taoists as the "Heart's Protector." It guards against anything that would invade or disturb one's consciousness and activates either the Virtue contained within the person or summons Heavenly Virtue to counterbalance any harmful energies.

2. Stomach 25, "The Heavenly Pivot" (two points/two dragons). It is thought that here is where Heaven and Earth meet in the body, since it is part of the body's center of gravity, just lateral to the navel. Gravity is seen as a force of Heaven, binding matter together and making all actions possible. The body must harmonize with this force from its center at Stomach 25.

   It is the influential point of the large intestine. The large intestine's energetic function is the same as its physiological function: to discharge that which is toxic to a person. This could mean waste from assimilating food, or it could mean the energy from a traumatic experience absorbed into a body, creating pain, disharmony, and disconnectedness from what is beneficial.

   In order to continue on the trajectory of one's personal evolution, when a trauma occurs and one is knocked off of one's path, it is necessary to pivot direction; in effect, this means to use the force of a trauma to propel one forward toward the next phase of evolution. After trauma occurs, it is sorted at "Dove Tail," the disharmony is discharged at "Heavenly Pivot," and the center of gravity in the person pivots and the person is propelled forward.

3. Stomach 32, "Prostrate Hare" (two points/dragons). The name comes from a Han Dynasty carving showing the Queen Mother of the West presiding over a number of figures, including a three-legged bird and a kneeling Rabbit, who offer her medicinal plants. The Rabbit is symbolic of the stomach, which takes things in (including experience), and the large intestine, which lets things go. The kneeling Rabbit is seen as both reverential of heavenly forces and as having respect for the divine plan.

4. Stomach 41, "Loosened Ravine" (two points/dragons). The image is seen in the Chinese character combination of *jie,* a slender instrument or blade made from the horn of an ox used to untie

or undo, to loosen or release, and *xi,* a ravine or depression in the earth, a place to discard what is not useful. It is located at the front of the ankle and is seen as returning to the earth what isn't needed to be regenerated, like waste is used to fertilize the ground to promote new growth. In one sense, this dragon may be seen as promoting new growth or providing firm ground on which to stand. The point is often used by itself to break long-standing habitual behavior that prevents one from providing sympathy and nourishment, both to one's self and to others.

FOR YOU:

Most practitioners should be familiar with seven dragons, so feel free to ask for it. Gianna reminds us that finding the right licensed practitioner can be like dating: You have to find the right match, so don't give up on the modality if you don't vibe with the practitioner. Begin finding the right person by asking friends and family for referrals. Your doctor might have suggestions as well.

If you do experience heightened emotions or panic attacks, in order to ground and calm yourself, Gianna suggests massaging the point between the eyebrows called yin tang, as well as a point on the bottom of your foot, under the ball of the foot closest to the arch, called Kidney 1. Zisser recommends pulling on and massaging your ears because the ears have all the acupressure points. You can also purchase ear seeds online and consult the NADA website (acudetox.com) for tutorials on how to apply them yourself. She also suggests rubbing the palm of your hand; applying pressure or tapping this point, known as Heart 8, will calm you down, as will pressing on the point known as Pericardium 6. Pericardium 6 is located about two thumb widths from your inner wrist crease on your thumb side.

Both Minka and Gianna emphasize the importance of nourishing, "predigested" foods for supporting the body in reharmonizing. Bone broths and soups in general are good to have because they support the spleen, an underappreciated organ in Western medicine. Chinese medicine practitioners believe the spleen is a filter for the blood and is responsible for separating the qi (energy) from our food and distributing it appropriately throughout the body. Foods that are naturally yellow or orange in color, such as yams and carrots, are also good to eat to boost the spleen. To help clear and drain the heart, Minka recommends bitter greens and mint tea. To maintain kidney health, eat a handful of walnuts (with the skin on) sauteed in sesame oil with a pinch of ground cloves and salted to taste.

Herbal remedies are also used in Chinese medicine to support the effects of acupuncture, and although it is best to work with a practitioner one-on-one, Minka suggests reishi as being a universally safe and helpful supplement unless you have a mushroom allergy. Reishi is good for digestion, calms the mind, and helps with sleep. Gianna recommends soothing herbal blends like boiled ginger, goji berries, licorice, and astragalus, an herb with many benefits. You can purchase many herbs in capsule or tincture form for under $10/bottle on iherb.com or Amazon if your local health food store doesn't carry them. If possible, go with a certified organic source.

Who is it right for? Wrong for?

There really isn't anybody who can't benefit from acupuncture. It is even safe for children and pregnant women. A licensed acupuncturist will work with you and your body to work out a safe and appropriate treatment plan.

GUA SHA

Gua sha is an ancient Chinese therapy used for healing and beautification. Using a smooth stone, the skin is scraped to release toxins, move lymph, and promote well-being. Gua sha can be used to supplement acupuncture and/or acupressure or on its own.

I discovered gua sha through Gianna. She is the cofounder of Wildling, a gua sha–based skin care company. I began practicing gua sha on my face a few times a week. After washing my face, I apply some facial oil and practice five movements, five to six times each, on each side of my face. The promise of "natural Botox" effects, lifting and firming, appealed to my vanity, and I did begin to see some positive results. It wasn't all vanity! When I would perform the gua sha, I noticed the calming effect the practice had on me. Also, Gianna had mentioned that gua sha on the neck and shoulders can help relieve stress, which piqued my curiosity further. Could gua sha be helpful with transmuting other symptoms of residual trauma?

When I posed this question to Gianna, she said: "Absolutely. Particularly when performed on the upper back. We store grief between the shoulder blades, so having someone work that area, as well as your neck and shoulders, will help to release grief." She also made sense of why gua sha is so calming to the nervous system by sharing that those micromovements on the face are reminiscent of how we used to groom each other as primates. Studies have also been done exploring the effectiveness of alternative therapies, such as gua sha, integrated with more traditional therapies, for treating PTSD in veterans and active service members. They have shown that these complementary therapies have a positive effect on patients' outcomes. These therapies allow for empowerment of patients by fostering greater interest and collaboration in their own healing, lessening of symptoms, and better stress management skills.[4]

FOR YOU:

Gua sha tools can be ordered online. The best tools are smooth stone, often jade, and have a few different angles with smooth edges, and sometimes one edge that looks like a comb, ideal for rubbing gently over fine lines. Holistic esthetician and Wildling Beauty cofounder Britta Plug offers this mini tutorial:[5]

1. Wash your face. Gua sha is best performed on clean skin primed with a serum or moisturizer so that the stone slides smoothly.

2. Angle the gua sha tool as close to parallel with your skin as possible (you don't want to dig the edge straight in like you're chopping), place the fingers of your free hand close to the tool's edge to provide some resistance, and then gently sweep the tool up and out toward the perimeter of your face. At the end of each stroke, give the tool a little extra wiggle to help release the tension (the edges of the face are chock-full of overworked muscle and ligament connections).

3. Repeat each stroke three times—you can build up to more
once you've learned your skin's tolerance, however, Plug says
not to exceed ten—concentrating on puff-prone areas such as
the cheeks and under the eyes.

Plug has many video tutorials and further tips on her website
Wildling Beauty. Wildling sells stones and gua sha kits for the body
as well as the face.

Who is it right for? Wrong for?

Gua sha should be avoided by those on blood thinners. If you have
a skin condition, you may want to consult with your dermatologist
before beginning gua sha. In general, keep your pressure light and
gentle on the face. Pressing too strongly can cause bruising. On the
body, you can use more vigorous pressure. If you're pregnant, avoid
scraping the tops of your shoulders and your belly.

QIGONG

Qigong, also known as chi gong or chi kung, is often a kind of moving meditation (though some forms are entirely still and primarily use breathwork
and intention), and is an important part of ancient Chinese medicine and
health promotion. It moves energy through the body in ways that bring the
body, mind, and spirit into better balance. Qigong master Ou Wen Wei explains that qigong has existed since the beginning of human history. He says
the purpose of qigong is to help people make adjustments to their physical
structures, minds, and emotions, and to help individuals make good daily
decisions by cultivating their heart and soul.

There is a great deal of poetry and metaphor in the explanation of
how and why it works. Because qigong postures, movements, and breathing patterns mimic recurrent patterns in nature, the qi (energy) in our
bodies comes into vibration with the universal flow of energy and therefore into the harmonious state and vibration in nature. Ou takes the
explanation of how it works deeper: "Practicing qigong helps us absorb
a kind and benevolent energy that has good effects on the whole person
when received. Modern science and technology don't fully understand
what exactly this energy is, but it has been scientifically detected and
measured." Studies reporting the beneficial results of qigong have been

conducted by such esteemed institutions as Harvard University and the Cleveland Clinic.[6]

Sometimes symptoms can be exacerbated or might appear after consistent qigong practice. I asked Ou why something good for us would make us feel worse. "When the new positive energy (qi) enters the body, it will make positive adjustments, improving body functions and assisting the body to come back into natural balance," he explains. Ou advises,

> I encourage my students to be persistent and to tolerate the discomfort that may occur when the body becomes sufficiently strong to make the necessary internal adjustments to bring the body into a state of harmony. If one is able to be persistent and tolerate the discomfort, then they may experience the positive results more quickly. However, if it becomes too intense, it is okay to take a break and to continue their practice when they feel ready.

Qigong teacher, Chinese medicine practitioner, and healer Paul Fraser shared his story about his triumph over a rare, malignant bone disease that followed him throughout his teen years. He was not expected to survive to adulthood but was physically, emotionally, and spiritually healed through qigong. This healing art both saved his life and changed the course of it entirely.

After being discharged from the hospital with a bleak prognosis, he stood on a train platform in excruciating pain and shrouded with depression. He saw a billboard for acupuncture from the train platform that led him to Chinese medicine practitioner and qigong master Tom Tam. After listening to Fraser's story of illness and pain, Tam told him he would treat him; if Fraser didn't feel better, he wouldn't have to pay.

Fraser felt himself pass into a healthy, normal physical state for about ten seconds after their first session. Because of that glimmer, he signed on with Tam for a six-week qigong training. Within those six weeks, Fraser says, "everything normalized."

After his body had healed, Fraser began having horrible nightmares, seeing himself as dead or dying: he had, after all, come back from the deep trauma of a terminal diagnosis before his young nervous system had even matured to adulthood. This is how Fraser explained this phenomenon: As energy moves through qigong practice, the residue of trauma moves with it. This can be painful at first, but ultimately, it helps bring positive energy to it and will transform it. The body holds the remedy for its own trauma, and through dedicated study and practice, your body can self-heal. "After about three or four months of practice, I could think the traumatic thoughts and not feel the associated feelings," he told me.

Fraser has dedicated his life to practicing and teaching qigong. He says qigong "didn't just give me my life back, it showed me how to live it."

I started following some of Fraser's qigong sequences online because I was having some neck and back pain (areas where typically stress and excess anxiety are held). Honestly, I wasn't expecting much, but it was worth a shot. Miraculously, with just a few minutes of some simple movements, I felt my pain go away! I also felt myself settle. Not sure if it was a fluke, I kept at it and kept noticing the positive benefits to my mind and body. Working with Fraser one-on-one via the phone and Zoom, I learned various qigong forms. Pangu shengong, created by Ou, is the practice I have woven into my daily routine. Since incorporating the practice into my life, I notice how much more patience, energy, and love I have, along with how I also seem to be magnetizing good and happy opportunities and situations faster and more easily.

· ·

FOR YOU:

Qigong training is widely available in larger metropolitan areas. Master Ou offers classes and sessions through his website pangu.org as well as many resources and more information. Fraser's book *Qi Gong: Rediscovering Our Humanity* offers a more in-depth, thorough, yet clear understanding of qigong. He also shares many tools (including qigong practice videos) on his website, paulfraserqigong.net. Another good reference book with very clear explanations was written by Fraser's second teacher, Yang Jwing-Ming, called *Chinese Qigong*. Ken Cohen's book *The Way of Qigong: The Art and Science of Chinese Energy Healing* is well written and clear as well. Daoist Gate is a website that offers some easy-to-follow streaming classes, and Yang's site, YMAA, has well-curated books, videos, and more on qigong.

Here are three movements Fraser shared that help to move and clear the unwanted residue of trauma. In his words, these moves "circulate the qi throughout the whole body; as the qi encounters the vibration of trauma, which has its own frequency relative to the event and one's perception and experience of it, the healthy qi will neutralize the trauma qi, rearrange and elevate its vibration into something that enhances life, or expel it."

Three Movements to Neutralize or Expel the Vibration of Trauma

1. Hold the palms in front of the chest about six inches apart, facing each other, relaxed, shoulders down. Imagine breathing in through the palms to the heart and down to the abdomen, filling it, and exhale through the soles of the feet, about three feet below the surface of the floor/ground, for six to twelve repetitions.

2. Extend the left arm, palm facing up, relaxed and with a moderate bend in the elbow, at about the height of your chest. Bringing the right palm to the center of your chest, still approximately six to eight centimeters away, trace a line from the center of the chest down the center of the interior part of the arm (this is the pericardium meridian) down to the left palm and extending beyond your fingertips. While tracing with the right palm, the left arm draws back until the right palm has passed the left fingertips. With the right arm now extended in front of the chest, turn it over so that the palm faces up. At the same time, turn over the left palm, bring it to face the center of the chest, then trace a line down the center of the right arm; the right arm draws back until the left palm passes the center of the palm and fingertips. As always, the key to this movement is keeping the tension out of the hands and arms. Leading the qi first through the left pericardium meridian and then through the right pericardium meridian counts as one repetition. Repeat this six to thirty-six times.

3. Slightly bend the knees (if you have knee problems, it's okay to do this upright, just not quite as effective), place palm over palm, resting on the abdomen, just below the navel; inhale to the abdomen, filling it, to where the palms meet, and exhale through the soles of the feet, imagining the breath three feet below the surface of the ground/floor.

If you are experiencing an acute panic attack or extreme anxiety, Ou suggests repeating the "password," the opening and closing lines of the pangu shengong practice if you practice that style, or simply continue to repeat the words "kindness and love" to yourself over and over, if you haven't learned that style yet. Both will help to calm and ground you.

Who is this right for? Wrong for?

"Soft"-style qigong is beneficial to everyone because the goal of these styles is to create greater health and harmony in the body and spirit. Soft styles restore optimal organ function and boost the immune system while also cultivating a stronger connection to the dao, the divine flow of the universe. Ou's pangu shengong would be considered a soft style and is safe and beneficial to everyone.

Ou cautions that there are many styles of qigong, and they all absorb different types of energy. Some styles can actually bring negative energy to the heart. "Hard"-style qigong usually consists of isometric exercises that mimic the actions of fighting, coordinated with concentrated breathing techniques. These hard styles were really designed for young men in the military and were not created for long-term practice because many of these warriors didn't live very long lives. Hard styles can be harmful, especially to women, and should not be practiced by anyone for a long time. Look for qigong classes and teachers that describe the work as calming and don't have special requirements or restrictions. If in doubt, ask!

In cases of psychosis, and other conditions prone to delusion, it is best to be closely monitored by a professional while engaging in these activities.

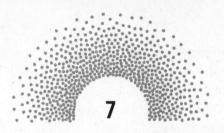

7

Let's Get Clinical

S ome therapies require the guidance and facilitation of a trained therapist or healer. Several of the therapies I cover in this chapter focus on
the intellectual, rational part of a person and have been scientifically
researched and their outcomes measured. Other therapies I outline are more
cutting edge, with less research behind them despite their significant allevia-
tion of symptoms. When we find therapeutic support with healers like those I
discuss here, we benefit from their extensive knowledge and experience in modalities that (for the most part) have substantial backing in scientific research.

EYE MOVEMENT DESENSITIZATION AND REPROCESSING THERAPY (EMDR)

EMDR was developed in 1987 by psychologist Francine Shapiro. Shapiro
discovered EMDR by synchronicity while walking in the park. She noticed
that as she was dwelling on some painful memories while rapidly moving
her eyes, she experienced marked relief from her distress.[1] After years of
observation and research, Shapiro realized that when her clients followed
the left-to-right movement of her raised finger with their eyes while recounting traumatic memories, they underwent a kind of reprogramming
in which the memories became less and less emotionally charged, a process
called desensitization. These clients would go from total terror at revisiting
these memories to little or no emotional response. I had EMDR myself and

share the common observation that before the therapy, your present self is still viscerally IN the memory; afterward, it's as though you are watching the memory as a movie from a safe and emotionally neutral distance.

Over the years, practitioners have recognized that the key to EMDR's effectiveness is *bilateral stimulation* (auditory, visual, or tactile stimuli that occur in a rhythmic left-right pattern), which can be achieved with eye movements, alternate tapping of hands on thighs or upper arms, or hand-held buzzers that vibrate alternately. With bilateral stimulation and skillful therapeutic guidance in recalling the traumatic memory, the client's connection to the memory of the event with a negative internal message—"I'm going to die"—is replaced with a positive truth: "I am strong; I survived." EMDR allows for the traumatic memories to be integrated into the person's experience, allowing for a more coherent body, mind, and spirit.

During the rapid eye movement (REM) period of our sleep cycles, many of the small traumas that occurred throughout the day are processed and cleared. EMDR practitioners' understanding is that the treatment mimics the REM cycle, and that is what effectively helps clear the larger trauma.

EMDR can be more effective than pharmaceutical drugs such as Prozac and Zoloft and can have more lasting effect than the drugs themselves.[2] The US Department of Veterans Affairs has approved EMDR as a treatment for PTSD in service members.

I walked into the therapist's office a complete mess two weeks after the mudslide. I had studied EMDR while earning my master's degree in psychology yet had never experienced it. It was the first therapy I tried because it came recommended by a close friend, a seasoned practitioner who assured me it would help. I wasn't sleeping because of nightmares and anxiety (Where would we live? Would my baby be okay? How would we pay for anything? We had just lost our greatest financial asset, our house, and insurance companies were saying they wouldn't step in because they don't cover "water damage" and "flooding"). And even if I was able to get to sleep in the first place, I had terrible poison oak rashes all over my legs that would wake me in the night with insatiable itchiness and burning. I was skeptical that EMDR would help a lot, and quickly, but I was desperate for relief.

We talked a bit about what was going on, and the therapist explained how the treatment would go for me. Keep in mind that the pacing, intensity and way the EMDR is used is tailored to each individual given their circumstances and window of tolerance. Per her directions, I held a buzzer in each hand that alternated buzzing to stimulate my bilateral brain connection while I recounted my memory of the mudslide in as graphic detail as I could recall, starting from waking up and jumping out of bed to seeing the mudslide careening toward us through the window. What was I aware of? What did I see? Hear? She involved all of my senses, making me recall the terrifying thunderous approach of the mudslide. She made me remember the earthy smell of the mud, which enveloped me and then trapped me—mud mixed with gas, sewage from ruptured septic tanks, walls of homes it had decimated and engulfed before reaching mine.

The first time I recounted the memory, I had trouble breathing. My heart was pounding in my chest. I felt like I wasn't really in my body. I cried. I had been responding this way in my daily life every time I told the story. I was being asked to tell it over and over by family, friends, insurance companies, and the Federal Emergency Management Agency (FEMA). I was being asked to tell it so often that I finally posted the story on Facebook so I wouldn't have to keep retraumatizing myself. However, in that first EMDR session, I told the story at least four times. Each time I told it while holding the buzzers, I felt a shift. Through the therapist's directives, I noticed how my changing language moved me from being a victim to being a strong survivor who had used her voice to awaken and save her family. My emotions leveled out, and my heart rate slowed down. My fear abated a little more each time I told the story. As we wrapped up the session, I felt immensely better than when I'd walked in, but I was still skeptical that anything had really changed.

That night, though, for the first time since the mudslide, I didn't have a nightmare. I started to notice that my trauma response had diminished. I was able to think more clearly and handle the details of my life more capably without feeling incapacitated. Everyone's progress will not be as rapid as mine was, but for me it was a profoundly helpful therapy.

I returned for a few more sessions. Each time, I felt steadier and more optimistic. Months later, as panic attacks emerged, I returned for more EMDR sessions. Return visits when trauma gets reactivated are part of the process for many.

....

FOR YOU:

The best way to find an EMDR-trained therapist is to ask your own therapist (if you are working with one) or friends for a referral.

Additionally, the EMDR International Association lists more than ten thousand EMDR-trained therapists around the world. If you are unable to work with a therapist in person, which I recommend trying first, you might try working with a therapist online using Zoom or FaceTime.

If working with a therapist is not an option, you can replicate the effects of bilateral stimulation at home. To be clear, you will not be practicing EMDR on yourself by yourself because this could be harmful, but through the practice of resource tapping you can achieve a similar benefit. Laurel Parnell's book *Tapping In: A Step-by-Step Guide to Activating Your Healing Resources Through Bilateral Stimulation* (Sounds True, 2008) is an excellent guide for what she calls resource tapping. Resource tapping uses simple bilateral stimulation to bring calm. Lucina Artigas developed this method in 1998 while working with survivors of Hurricane Pauline in Acapulco, Mexico. It has become a widely used and accepted practice for clinicians working with survivors of human-caused and natural catastrophes. It is a quick and easy form of calming self-care that can be done anywhere.

Try this:

1. Close your eyes. Place one hand on each thigh or cross your arms over your chest in a "butterfly" posture with each hand on the opposite upper arm.

2. Think of a time you felt calm and strong or picture a real or imaginary peaceful place. See and sense as many details as possible: temperature, sounds, smells, sights.

3. After you have a positive feeling in your body, begin to tap your fingers, alternating right and left, on your thighs or upper arms. (You can even do this by alternately tapping the toes on your right and left sides if you're trying to be subtle.) Aim for about six to twelve taps, with twelve as the maximum.

You can also practice this method by scrunching your toes, alternating right and left, if you are in a public place. In fact, during one of my panic attacks at a big luncheon where I was up front and center, I tapped my feet back and forth on the floor to calm myself down. I didn't even realize I was activating bilateral stimulation, yet I was, and it worked! Tapping your thighs with your hands is also an option; I've often done this on an airplane.

Who is it right for? Wrong for?

EMDR is an excellent therapy for recent, acute traumatic events. It's also a good option for anyone reluctant or unable to speak about their trauma. EMDR can be helpful even if you are not verbal during the therapy; it is about your observation of your traumatic memories in a new way, not about the verbal exchange with a practitioner.

Rendy Freeman, who has been practicing EMDR for almost twenty years, shares: "Often, when you clear one trauma, it tends to clear other incidents and situations." In this way, it can also help mitigate negative beliefs formed as a result of childhood abuse. When you target a certain traumatic incident, you can clear trauma from chronic abuse; for example, using EMDR to focus on a time when a hypercritical parent was verbally abusive might heal you of negative beliefs born of that abuse. Habitual self-talk around not being "good enough" or being unable to do anything right can linger for decades after it has come in through unkind words from a parent. EMDR, even regarding a different trauma, can create a welcome shift by releasing residue from a constellation of other traumas as well. Although EMDR is an incredible tool for alleviating the aftereffects of trauma, it is not appropriate for everyone; your therapist or doctor can let you know if it will be helpful given the nature of your trauma and where you are on your healing journey.

CRANIOSACRAL THERAPY (CST)

Sarah Rebstock, craniosacral and massage therapist, offered me a complimentary session through a friend who had told her what I had recently been through. Her tiny therapy room in a yoga studio was dim and smelled like incense and patchouli. She was barefoot and not wearing any makeup, hair in braids, sweet, welcoming, and nurturing. It was a week or so after the mudslide, and it was such a relief and a comfort to lie there, receive, and relax that I actually fell into a restorative sleep, something that had been eluding me post-mudslide.

As with the EMDR, the session brought me instantaneous relief that endured for a while. It felt as though my brain went into a deeper state where healing actually occurs, free from the chatter of the thinking brain. The "rational/thinking" brain was quieted, and I was in a meditative dream state when I wasn't asleep. I felt like Rebstock helped my brain and my body let go of the gripping hypervigilance that can persist after a trauma. The amygdala, the part of the brain that senses threat, is on high alert following a trauma, and my amygdala needed to be told to relax and let go because I was no longer in danger.

The treatment itself consists of a full-body massage that ends with the practitioner sort of cradling your head. Pressing gently on parts of the neck and skull to induce relaxation and release, or as Rebstock explains it, "meeting a person with what I've named 'the touch of observation.' At this point I am not trying to manipulate or change anything yet. I simply land, and ask, 'What is the tissue doing/trying to show me; what is the most acute thing I'm noticing; what is the most subtle/almost imperceptible thing?'"

She explains that she silently introduces herself to the inner healer of the client, offering her service, stating her boundaries, and inviting that part of the client to show her what it needs. The Upledger Institute, founded by John Upledger, one of the world's foremost craniosacral experts, calls this initial phase *blending and melding*. With trauma, this phase usually takes longer, Rebstock explains, not because it is harder to discern what is going on in the body but to build trust, gently allow the client's central nervous system to regulate to your presence and touch, and let the tissue invite you in at its own pace. Being patient here is key. Force nothing. Rebstock emphasizes that the practitioner being invited is necessary. This recognizes and honors the bodily autonomy of the client, and for a traumatized body this is even more important.

Rebstock sheds light on what she experiences in working with the client:

> Once invited, you follow the thread. For every CST practitioner I'm
> sure it's different. What I feel is usually felt in my hands, except for
> when my body cues me that I'm in the right spot and that I need to
> pause and await a deeper invitation. This manifests as a rush of chills
> over my face and a drop in my sternum to my diaphragm (a sense
> of "landing deeper"), the tissue feels expectant, starts up a therapeutic
> pulse that often gets more rapid, heat is released, and then the pulse
> peaks and the tissue starts to change, often softening and spreading,
> or pulling you immediately into the next place that needs to release,
> maybe just next to the initial spot. Often tissue will unwind, assuming

the same position that it was in when the trauma occurred. This can look like a whole body moving (coming off the table in some cases) or a joint moving itself into a position to allow the tissue to release and change. Sometimes after a local release (specific to a spot) there will be a global integration (whole body change). This can be subtle or dramatic, depending on the session. This work often accesses the emotional experience of the releases as well as the physical. After all, we are one holistic system living a complex, layered experience continuously. When the work starts to integrate on the levels where the physical and emotional meet, we often start to speak, both to determine that we are still within the client's boundaries and consent, and also to mirror back their experience to allow the work to continue and deepen.

....

FOR YOU:

Again, like some of the other therapies that don't require speech, CST is a great therapy to work with soon after a trauma or if you don't feel comfortable verbalizing. Find a practitioner through the Upledger Institute (upledgerclinic.com), one of the leading craniosacral institutions. You can also find someone through word of mouth or a referral, which is how I met Rebstock. If you happen to be in Santa Barbara, she is an angel on earth, and I would recommend her wholeheartedly: sarahrebstock.com.

As pricing varies, research and call facilities and practitioners in your area.

Who is it right for? Wrong for?
CST is not an appropriate treatment for those suffering from acute traumatic brain injury, recent skull fracture, brain tumors, acute stroke, acute cerebral hemorrhage, aneurysm, or any acute cerebral vascular condition or active bleeding. As always, if you are unsure if CST is a good fit for you, consult with a doctor. If you are suffering from issues about someone touching your body, with a trusted practitioner, this sort of treatment might serve as a bridge to helping you reclaim your body and its physical sensations.

NEUROLINGUISTIC PROGRAMMING (NLP)

Neurolinguistic programming (NLP) is a psychotherapy technique that focuses on patterns and styles of communication. It addresses how to disrupt and undo unhealthy programs and patterns we run in our brains in order to release, heal, and reprogram our brains in a healthy way. NLP was formulated in the 1970s by linguist John Grinder and scientist and mathematician Richard Bandler, who focused their work on people who had overcome difficulties successfully rather than on people in crisis.

NLP therapy consists of working with eye movements, as with EMDR, in order to move an issue through a particular cortex of the brain. Kim Vincent, NLP practitioner, explains that after a trauma or debilitating event, our brains can get stuck in a traumatic loop. This loop manifests either visually in that we experience flashbacks, auditorily in that we are saying something to ourselves and/or noises are triggering us, or kinesthetically in that we feel the residual effects of the event in our bodies. The eye movements help to scramble these loops, desensitizing us to the memory. This allows more space around the memory, promoting healing and the formation of new neural pathways.

I had heard about Vincent through a friend who had seen the practitioner for her fear of flying. My friend had undergone NLP with Vincent, and then participated in ongoing therapy that she found hard to describe, but it was clearly effective because she boarded a plane with minimal anxiety for her anniversary trip a few months later. She mentioned that it was apparently very helpful for trauma as well. The problem was that Vincent was located almost an hour away, in the bucolic hippie town of Ojai. I wasn't sure when I could commit that amount of time to trying out a new healing method.

And then I really committed. I signed up for a retreat in Ojai right around the first anniversary of the mudslide. It seemed like a good time to retreat, restore, and heal. I contacted Vincent for a session, and lo and behold, she was one of the speakers at the retreat! We got to spend time together during the retreat, which made our first session all the more powerful and useful for me. I've seen her many times since for trauma help as well as for major life transitions that followed my healing and integration of my lessons learned.

We always sit and chat for a bit, and Vincent offers me a cup of tea. I haven't told you she is British. She is also blonde, with sparkly eyes and a warm, accepting persona that makes you feel safe and seen—yet she can also get down to business when it's time. We have our tea and chat, and then we really laser focus in on the issue we're addressing that day. We addressed my massive fear first, particularly about storms, perfect because it actually stormed the entire time we were on the retreat, and evacuations were being ordered back in Montecito. Retriggering, to say the least!

Vincent had me stand up and asked me if I was ready to do some work. It always feels a bit hard to cheerfully say, "I am!" But I do. The first time I was skeptical about whether I was going to feel anything—if it could really work to follow her finger with my eyes, "rewind" the memory, and have it release its hold on me. But it worked. And it worked for days and weeks thereafter. Sometimes even when things "work" on a spiritual or emotional level, our doubting human minds want "proof." Vincent explained to me that rewinding the movie reel of our trauma we have on a loop "disrupts the imprint of the experience and resets the brain so that the body can have a different response to the memory and heal."

It was another perfect coincidence that one day when I went to see Vincent for a session, I was suffering from allergies. I have never in my life had allergies until I moved to Santa Barbara, where everything thrives and blooms and grows. I had been reluctantly taking Claritin to stave off the headache, nasal drip, and brain fog. I mentioned this to Vincent, who said, "Your body is currently perceiving something as a threat that isn't dangerous and having a reaction to it. Shall we get rid of these allergies?" She warned me it could take a couple of sessions. We hopped up, and standing next to me, she asked me to picture myself in an open-air house in a field full of grasses and trees and blooms all loaded with pollen and to see myself frolicking in all of this pollen, coated in it and not having any reaction to it. She asked me to follow her finger with my eyes, this way and that and round and round, and then I took a step back, and I have not had to take a Claritin ever since! Allergies were gone—poof!

In addition to the eye movements and rewinding the unhelpful movies of our past, Vincent employs shaking between eye movements to release the trauma on a cellular level, allowing for the body to reset and recalibrate. She shared that while living in England, she would watch the ducks sometimes get into it with each other, and after their scuffle, they would waddle away and shake it off. As human beings, we don't feel the freedom to have this very natural response, and so instead we freeze, locking the adrenaline into our bodies.

Vincent also consciously employs humor in her sessions as a way to distract the brain, allowing it to reset, and also as a way to change the emotional state around the trauma and healing. It is easier to work with and clear a trauma when we are in an elevated emotional state. Vincent emphasizes the importance of clearing trauma on all levels, including energetically. We can heal and understand something intellectually, but if we don't clear the energetic frequency of the event, the trauma still exists in our energetic field. This is especially detrimental because that frequency of fear and trauma attracts more trauma, given that frequencies attract and draw to them similar frequencies. So we must clear ourselves energetically. You can do this with an energy healer, but we can also energetically clear ourselves through meditation, qigong, and some of the other tools I explain in this book.

Vincent believes in the importance of healing holistically, especially because we don't want to create what she refers to as future traumatic stress syndrome (FTSD). Our lingering fear and anxiety would create a future traumatic situation that doesn't yet exist, yet we would respond and experience this made-up future trauma as if it had already happened. We might equate FTSD with panic attacks.

• •

FOR YOU:

Vincent recommends certified NLP practitioners who have trained in Tim and Kris Hallbom's NLP Institute of California's (nlpca.com) certification program. It's so important to find someone you resonate with and trust. The NLP Institute of California website is a good resource. Vincent also reminds us, "You are living proof that you survive everything." You have survived, and now through resetting the brain and body, you heal the soul, allowing for learning and integration. And you can thrive.

Who is it right for? Wrong for?
NLP is potentially beneficial for everyone. It is a particularly good therapy for grounding and stabilization because often during a traumatic event our natural response is to move up and out of our bodies, energetically speaking. We "leave" our bodies because what is happening is too scary, painful, or intense to stay present. NLP helps to bring us back into our bodies so that we can heal, clear our trauma, and create from a stable place.

PHARMACOLOGY

I have always been a little afraid of drugs after an experience with marijuana at the age of eighteen that left me feeling out of control, like I was spinning, and nauseated. While my other friends were giggling and having the time of their lives, I was in the fetal position praying for the sensation to end. So, having avoided drugs my entire adult life, other than alcohol, which I manage and enjoy responsibly, I had some trepidation about exploring some of the drug therapies for PTSD. As I did not personally take them and this book is an exploration of more alternative therapies, I'm not covering SSRIs, SNRIs, or mood stabilizing drugs. With the guidance and recommendation of a doctor, they can be a great option for some people.

My own journey led me to research and prepare myself to try 3,4-methylenedioxy-N-methylamphetamine (MDMA) therapy just before Covid-19 hit. MDMA, otherwise known as ecstasy, is known to induce great feelings of warmth and love by flooding the brain with serotonin, a neurotransmitter in the brain responsible for making us feel good. I had interviewed two different therapists and found one in Santa Barbara with whom a friend had had wonderful experiences and with whom I felt really comfortable. Just as we were going to begin our preparatory sessions, California was ordered to lock down because of Covid-19, and my plans were thwarted.

About a year later, at a socially distanced lunch outside, I met a woman with whom I instantly connected. We had begun talking about this book and all of my research when she interjected that I had to meet her husband, a psychiatrist who had been doing ketamine therapy for years with incredible results.

Ketamine Therapy

I had a one-hour consultation with her husband, Dr. Jeff Becker, whose practice focuses on neuropsychiatry and functional medicine, and we talked about my history and my goal for working with him. After listening and asking some questions, he said he thought ketamine therapy would be beneficial for me. He explained that ketamine, the only legal psychedelic, is considered both gentle and powerful, so much so it's actually used in hospitals as an anesthetic for children. He loves working with it because the dosing is precise, unlike that of other psychedelics found in nature, such as mushrooms, with which you never know how much you are getting or giving. He also said that ketamine is a very "yin" drug, meaning that it is gentle in engendering sensations that want to be brought to your attention, as opposed to mushrooms, which Becker referred to as a "warrior sun psychedelic," with a very yang, "in-your-face" energy. Mushrooms *make* you see what needs to be seen and force you to burn it into your consciousness, whereas ketamine allows you to observe and integrate more at your own pace and comfort level. From my research, I knew that ketamine therapy was effective for treating depression and suicidal ideation, both of which I did not have, so I asked Becker more pointedly about treating PTSD.

Becker related experiences from a multitude of clients suffering from PTSD, saying that the ketamine allowed the individuals to see themselves and the traumatic events as somehow no longer personal. It was as if the ketamine allowed them to zoom out, recognize our interconnected experiences, and see that what had occurred was not personal but happened universally.

Ketamine works by disassembling neural networks in our mind, whose default mode, the executive and salience networks, ascribe significance to events and our sense of identity. Becker explains that on ketamine, while these networks are quieted, other neurons are able to connect with each other. He likened it to cliques: Instead of all the cheerleaders only talking to each other, the musicians hanging out only with each other, or the debate club members interacting only with each other, everyone is talking to everyone. Ketamine allows us to access our latent inner resources.

The shift in frequencies in the brain when ketamine is administered has been studied and documented. The frequencies of the brain are:

- delta, the slowest and the state we are in when we are in a deep sleep

- theta, a dreamlike, daydreaming state

- alpha, referred to as a Zen state, when we are calm and alert, ready to take action but not active

- beta, the multitasking, active, doing state

- gamma, the highest and fastest frequency, responsible for higher consciousness, a state of *knowing*

Most of us spend much of our time going between beta and theta states, working really hard, problem solving, and then daydreaming. On ketamine, all of the other frequency states are diminished except gamma, which goes way up and becomes more universalized rather than localized. These high gamma levels indicate what we already know: That ketamine allows us to experience a higher state of consciousness, to become aware of the universal I—the I who is observing the thinking I, the I who is connected to all.

Propranolol (Beta-Blockers)

To prepare for the ketamine therapy, Becker asked if anyone had prescribed propranolol for me after the mudslide. No, I didn't know what that was. Propranolol is a beta-blocker and blood pressure medicine, but it is also prescribed to help mitigate hyperactive fear responses, even in children. These panicky moments can lead to the proliferation of more fear and long-term changes in the brain that hardwire reactivity. This kind of fear is extremely common after a traumatic event because our amygdala (the part of the brain responsible for activating our fight/flight/freeze response) has been alerted, releasing cortisol and adrenaline to propel us to safety and away from the threat. The problem is when the amygdala doesn't turn off, which it naturally doesn't for about thirty days following a trauma. So the fear response is heightened and, in some people, actually keeps escalating.

Becker explained that the body remembers the flood of adrenaline and cortisol that helped us get to safety from the previous trauma. In the aftermath of the event, there can be changes that cause the brain to release *more* adrenaline and cortisol the next time a situation reminds us of the trauma, thinking that this time it will get us out of there faster, better, more safely. Evidence has shown that propranolol can block the consolidation, or learning, of these fear responses. It can help mitigate the changes that escalate posttraumatic fear responses. In other words, it might help block the development of PTSD. Someone who develops panic attacks while driving after experiencing a car accident could take a beta-blocker and drive with less of a fear response. It can help to break the cycle.

Propranolol is also very helpful in overcoming phobias. By blocking the adrenaline the phobia triggers, the person moves through the event with less activation. The fear response is blocked, and the trigger mechanisms don't "reconsolidate," meaning the fear doesn't build upon itself. You can take it preemptively, before an event known to elicit fear or while you are experiencing a fear response. For example, someone with a fear of flying can take a beta-blocker before the flight and unlearn the fear of flying by noticing that it wasn't scary to fly. It wasn't scary because the adrenaline was "blocked," and the association has been broken because the fear receptors in the brain have been blocked. The experience of flying while unafraid has created a new reality and new neural pathways, unwinding the old fear-based response. Unfortunately, sedatives have no such magic. People who take Xanax or another type of sedative before they fly aren't getting to the root cause of the fear. Propranolol helps us unlearn the fear response rather than masking it.

So, Becker gave me a prescription for propranolol, but he pointed out that low blood pressure is common in many women who have experienced trauma, as with me. He had me test a low dose of the beta-blocker to make sure I didn't feel lightheaded or pass out, then had me take one and drive around Montecito, where the mudslide occurred, to begin neutralizing my fear response. He also said I should take one about an hour before the first ketamine treatment, to help me relax into the treatment, so that I wouldn't fight the feelings of losing control. I was also instructed not to eat or drink for four hours before the treatment to avoid stomach upset.

We discussed the fact that he would inject an antinausea drug in one upper arm, then deliver the ketamine in three shots to the other arm. This was a way for us to be sure the dosing felt right and that I was doing okay before proceeding. It was also a way for me to share any images or thoughts with him as I became more lucid between "trips." Because ketamine has a very short half-life, meaning that its effects wear off quickly, each experience would last about fifteen to twenty minutes. He shared that music would enhance the experience and give it form, suggesting I could put together a playlist or that he could choose the music. To start, he recommended warm pieces mostly without lyrics, noting that tastes vary; some people prefer electronica with a beat, and others resonate more with new age pieces or classical music with real strings. He pointed to online resources developed by Mendel Kalen for more nuanced understanding of the value of music to psychedelic medicine.

The day of my first ketamine treatment, I was excited and also a little bit nervous. I journaled, giving thanks in my morning meeting (see chapter 8) for my gentle, yet profound, transcendent healing experience. I skipped my exercise routine, sensing that conserving my physical energy might be a good idea. I had Lucy pick me up because driving is not permitted for the several hours following a ketamine treatment, and we had a quiet lunch of soup and salad and chatted about my hopes for what the therapy would allow for me to uncover and integrate. I took the propranolol after lunch and felt fine, if a bit more relaxed. She dropped me off, promising to be back about two hours later, and wished me luck.

Becker welcomed me into his office in a California bungalow in downtown Santa Barbara. There was the usual couch with two chairs you imagine in a therapist's office. There was a retro-cool art lamp, one of many he started making in medical school, with gradations of oranges, greens, yellows, and other colors that illuminated the facing couch and bookshelves lined with books on lysergic acid diethylamide (LSD) therapy, meditation, and mind mapping. Becker gave me a shot of Zofran, an antinausea drug, right off the bat to give it enough time to kick in, then went through the protocol we were going to follow, discussing dosing and my hopes for the experience. Because it was my first time, and we weren't sure about my sensitivity, he recommended we start with a lower dose, and then we could ramp it up for the following two injections if I felt like I wanted to.

I settled into the leather reclining chair with my feet propped up on an ottoman, Becker covered me with a blanket, and I donned my eye mask, which he had recommended I wear. Swabbing my right upper arm, he injected the first dose, letting me know it would start to take effect in about five minutes, and we were off . . .

I had a pleasant sensation of falling, and my surroundings felt textural, like a fuzzy sweater or velvet. I didn't have a sense of my body anymore, but I had the sensation of warmth. I felt like there was a veil I wanted to see behind, blackness with bits of red swirling, but I couldn't see behind it. Apparently, I said to Becker, "This isn't scary at all. It's lovely. I feel like I'm floating." After the first shot was wearing off, Becker asked how I was doing, and I said that I wanted to feel and to see more; I was still somewhat aware of the room. So he agreed I needed a larger dose the second time, injected it, and I was off again. And was I ever!

The sensations intensified, and I was seeing kaleidoscopic effects, almost like colored oil in water, a lava lamp, something like that. And then I had a thought (or did I?) about addressing being molested at the age of seven, and should I look at that? And then I was sort of watching a version of the scene. I was outside of it, and then out of the blackness to the right of the scene, all these fragments started swirling together to form a large gorilla's face looking right at me, the me observing. At first, I wondered if I should be afraid of the gorilla, but I knew even as I was asking myself that question that this was a loving presence, and I wasn't afraid. And then I watched as the gorilla turned and whisked that little girl right out of that scene and away from that man. And then we were off again. And I was a more grown-up version of myself, although I didn't really have a body—I had really long flowing hair, and I was on the back of a beautiful white horse. We were flying, and I knew this was Pegasus, and I was on his back. He looked back at me, and I felt such love. It felt like a promise of love in my life here to fiercely guard me, protect me, and help me to fly.

After the third dose, which Becker upped a little more because I still had a sensation of wanting to see more, "see behind the curtain," the effects of floating in space, swimming through dark warm water, and looking through colored seaweed were pervasive. As I felt myself "rising to the surface," I asked the question (or again, did I?), "Is there anything else you (not sure who the you is) want me to see?" Almost immediately, it felt like I was ushered by strong angel wings to a perspective where I was watching the mudslide from far away as if it were one of those Renaissance oil paintings. And what I saw were beautiful, golden-winged angels in effect pouring the mud down that mountain. And while they were pouring it down, they were also reaching down and pulling souls up and out of it to them. It's as if I were watching from a peaceful, warm place far away, as if I were over the Pacific Ocean looking toward the mountains of Montecito. There was such peace, love, and understanding in this image.

After I came back to a more normal state of mind and into Becker's office, I felt a little groggy, as if I had awoken from a deep sleep. We chatted for a bit about my experience and the symbols that came up during the session. Although I felt "out of it," I can mostly recall our conversation. He pointed out that it was nice that the fierce protective gorilla part of myself showed up to protect that little girl. I appreciated this interpretation because I had thought of the gorilla as outside of myself, when really the experience was showing me a strong part of myself. This plays back into the theme of integrating our experiences, all of them, and also all of the various aspects of ourselves, through these healing modalities.

In the hours that followed, I felt like a mellower version of myself, with gentle epiphanies continuing to bubble up. The relaxed and appreciative state continued, and I was able to see a deeper, more intricate beauty in the people and nature around me. It was almost as if the ketamine sharpened my focus on the beautiful aspects of life, while at the same time it turned down the volume on the anxieties in me. I felt like myself, but a calmer and more insightful version. I also continue to have cathartic and healing "aha!" moments that have helped to clarify situations, relationships, and long-standing emotions and responses.

I asked Becker about these changes before my second session, and he explained that the ketamine does allow for new neural pathways to form. Neurons that normally don't have a chance to communicate with each other can experience connection during the session. Research has shown new dendritic densities and connections in the brain following ketamine treatments. This is exciting because it means participants' brains are being rewired, something scientists like to call *neuroplasticity*, or the brain's ability to change. Becker described the ketamine as creating "windows of opportunity" that allow for new experiences and reemergence of the true self as the trauma is integrated. These new experiences help create and reinforce the neural pathways of a healthy, whole identity. And, he said that if the benefits fade over time, or a challenging life event happens that triggers a retreat, a ketamine booster can help to process in real time, allowing a return to self more quickly.

I had three ketamine treatments to address my lingering anxiety and stress responses after the mudslide and to clean up some of the old gunk from childhood. Each one was healing, cathartic, and rather wondrous. It is a treatment I would absolutely revisit should something else come up to be cleared.

MDMA Therapy

I did wind up experimenting with MDMA therapy a few months after the ketamine therapy. MDMA allowed me to speak about, process, and reflect on my traumatic experiences, including the mudslide and instances of sexual abuse from my childhood, from a place of loving acceptance. The acceptance was of myself, how I survived and handled those situations, while experiencing them and then afterward.

Unlike on the ketamine, on the MDMA I was totally lucid and aware of my body and surroundings and didn't experience any visions not in my three-dimensional reality. The effect of the MDMA was more of exaggerating the beauty of my surroundings and of life in general. Light, color, and sound were more defined and pleasing, physical touch was heightened, and nature was more exhilarating. Similar to the ketamine effect of zooming out, I felt the same acceptance of the traumatic experiences, and when talking and reflecting on them in the MDMA-induced state, I experienced a sense of allowing. Some part of me allowed those experiences to integrate despite the fact that I had shoved them firmly off to the side as scary and harmful. I had relegated them to some island like Alcatraz in me, yet not of me. With the help of the MDMA and guided therapy, I felt a profound appreciation for life, all of my experiences, and the interconnectedness of all beings and circumstances. While in this state, I had an awareness that the mudslide was no longer haunting me. I felt quite resolved about it, like it was complete.

What did make me cry while thinking about the sexual abuse from my childhood was a lingering sense that I had somehow pulled these men and experiences to me, and then realizing there was no way that was possible. Nothing I had done as a seven-year-old child, a thirteen-year-old girl, and then an eighteen-year-old young woman had made these men do what they did. I realized I was just the little girl who happened to be "in front of them." I recognized that it was actually so impersonal, that there wasn't anything I did or could have done, and that just as the mudslide was a force of nature, a force of nature had moved through those men, and I was in their path. I felt compassion for these men because I believed they were acting out of an absence of love in their lives and that their acts of abuse were an attempt to fill that void. I forgave them for *me*, to untether myself from these murky feelings of shame and guilt that had been following me, lurking in my shadows for decades. I also had an expansive sense that *this*, "this" being a state free of judgment and limitation, is always present, and yet we have been so programmed to work against it, to not trust it, to place constraints and restraints on it and ourselves, that we don't access it.

MDMA was formulated by Merck scientists in 1912. Therapists started using it in the 1970s with profound results, yet it was outlawed in 1985 when it became a popular recreational drug otherwise known as ecstasy or Molly.[3] In the past few years, MDMA has once again been championed for its incredible benefits in therapy, especially in the treatment of PTSD and depression. MDMA elevates serotonin, oxytocin, and dopamine, all "feel-good" chemicals. With the levels of these chemicals elevated, feelings of love, compassion, and trust are heightened. Most compelling is the discovery that MDMA might help return the adult brain to the more malleable brain of childhood. This time in childhood, referred to by neuroscientists as the *critical period*, is when the brain has the superior ability to make new memories and store them.[4] This would indicate that MDMA might help with neuroplasticity and, in particular, rewriting traumatic memory so that it is no longer traumatic.

FOR YOU:

Propranolol

Propranolol was originally approved as a blood pressure medication and is now classified as a beta-blocker. Becker says it might be helpful for anyone severely traumatized because it blocks the adrenaline the brain releases when a fear response is triggered. Propranolol can be taken soon after a traumatic event to help avoid building a long-lasting adrenaline response that allows fears to proliferate. It can also be taken preemptively if you know you will be in a stressful or triggering situation. Finally, it can be taken after an unanticipated fear arises, specifically to help stop the ratcheting up of the process in the days that follow. Propranolol requires a prescription from a doctor or a nurse practitioner, but it is unscheduled and non-habit-forming. If you take it many times a day for a long time, you should taper off it, but otherwise there is no danger in taking it as needed in this way. Becker says that because propranolol can lower blood pressure and slow pulse, sometimes people can get dizzy if they stand up too quickly. People should start with a low dose (e.g., 10 mg) and only increase if they don't have this sensitivity. Generally doses from 10 to 40 mg are well tolerated.

Ketamine therapy

I asked Becker who might be good candidates for ketamine-assisted psychotherapy (KAP). He said simply, "Anybody trying to move past the haunting of their history that is keeping them from fully owning their life might find it helpful." He discussed appropriate screening and consent and emphasized the helpfulness of ketamine in processing trauma. He also made sure I understood that ketamine can be delivered intravenously and in lozenge form and that the protocol I experienced might be done differently in other offices. I found it one of the most powerful tools for me in healing from the traumas of the mudslide and of childhood sexual abuse as well as helping me through my divorce.

To find a reputable ketamine therapy provider, you can consult the Kriya Institute (kriyainstitute.com). It was founded by Raquel Bennett, a true pioneer and champion of using ketamine in therapeutic settings. The website has many articles and resources, including a list of approved providers. The American Society of Ketamine Practitioners (ASKP) is another excellent resource for learning more about ketamine therapy. It provides a directory of ketamine practitioners and is considered the governing body for clinical use of ketamine in mental health treatment in the United States.

Before your first ketamine session, be sure not to eat or drink for approximately four hours beforehand because the ketamine can upset your stomach. Becker gave me an injection of the antinausea drug Zofran about twenty to thirty minutes prior to administering the ketamine. He also had me take propranolol an hour before the session so that my adrenaline levels would remain in check because ketamine can be stimulating. He said the propranolol is a "soft call," meaning it can be included or not depending on the person and the therapy. Wear comfortable clothes and preferably a shirt where the practitioner can access your upper arm if they will be injecting the ketamine or doing an infusion.

Following your session, be sure to have someone pick you up, and give yourself several hours to relax, integrate, and journal what came up during the session. Be aware and record what continues to come up for you in the days that follow. Becker says to take special note of symbolism that appears during your experience and in the days afterward. Jungian psychologist Edward Edinger thought of symbols as offerings from the deep self, pointing toward primary truth.

> A symbol . . . is an image or representation which points to something essentially unknown, a mystery. A sign communicates abstract, objective meaning whereas a symbol conveys living, subjective meaning. A symbol has a subjective dynamism which exerts a powerful attraction and fascination on the individual. It is a living, organic entity which acts as a releaser and transformer of psychic energy. We can thus say a sign is dead, but a symbol is alive. Symbols are spontaneous products of the archetypal psyche. One cannot manufacture a symbol, one can only discover it. Symbols are carriers of psychic energy. This is why it is

proper to consider them as something alive. They transmit to the ego, either consciously or unconsciously, life energy which supports, guides, and motivates the individual.[5]

Carl Jung thought of symbols as the "real thing" and referred to signs and words as mere placeholders. For me, the symbols of the fierce and protective gorilla represented a needed aspect of myself; Pegasus represented true love and freedom; and the golden angels were the divine aspect of the universe showing me there is ultimately no bad or good, no duality, but everything is divine. Everything just *is*.

Prazosin

I asked Becker if there was anything else he might recommend to help alleviate the distressing symptoms that can linger in the wake of a major transition or traumatic event. He mentioned Prazosin, interestingly another high blood pressure medication that can help with sleep. It works by blocking certain receptors in the brain and has the effect of decreasing dreaming and nightmares. I never took Prazosin, but from my own experience, lack of sleep exacerbates feelings of being out of control, ungrounded, and unwell. We need deep sleep to reset, recalibrate, integrate, and reboot.

MDMA therapy

MDMA is still classified as an illegal drug. There are promising studies pointing to its efficacy in treating PTSD, and the hope is that it might be legalized by 2023. It can be used safely with positive results in the right setting with the correct dose; however, things can go wrong if it is used without reverence. Consult with your doctor before beginning any kind of psychedelic therapy. The Multidisciplinary Association of Psychedelic Study (MAPS) is a great resource. Founded in 1986 by Rick Doblin, MAPS fund-raises, educates, and advocates for the beneficial use of psychedelic therapies.

Who is it right for? Wrong for?

Again, I am not a doctor, and any time you are considering taking drugs, speaking to and working with a doctor about your unique biology and condition is critical to ensuring the path forward for you is healthy, helpful, and right for you.

Propranolol

If you have low blood pressure, be mindful of taking propranolol for the first few times. Try a small dose in an environment where you don't stand up abruptly, drive, and so forth. Propranolol might potentially help anyone with strong fear reactions and/or phobias.

Ketamine therapy

Anyone suffering from unresolved trauma, symptoms of PTSD, depression, and/or thoughts of suicide can be a candidate for ketamine therapy. Even if there isn't a specific significant trauma to resolve, the drug can help offer perspective and relief. It is one of the most effective treatments for suicidality and has been shown to significantly help with treatment-resistant depression.

Ketamine is generally not recommended for individuals with schizophrenia because it has been shown to reactivate psychosis in some cases. It can be used in bipolar disorder when depression is the issue, but caution should be exercised because some practitioners believe it might be capable of triggering mania. As with all the recommendations I make in this book, I must offer this disclaimer acknowledging that you understand that I am not liable for any personal injury arising from ketamine therapy or any of the other pharmaceuticals mentioned here. Be sure to go over any and all concerns you have with your doctor.

Prazosin

You might want to ask about prazosin if you are having trouble sleeping in the context of bad dreams and flashbacks related to trauma. If your sleep is interrupted by traumatic nightmares, this medication can be a way to quiet the storm without use of sedatives such as Ativan or Klonopin, which can cause dependence if abused. Again, be aware and tell your doctor if you have low blood pressure before taking prazosin, and, as Becker says, "start low and go slow."

MDMA therapy

Consult with your doctor before embarking on MDMA therapy. It has been shown to be highly beneficial to those struggling with PTSD, depression, and anxiety. According to Rachel Yehuda, director of Mt. Sinai's Traumatic Stress Studies Department, there can be some contraindications, so undergoing a physical clearance with a physician is recommended.

SUPPORT GROUPS

I never attended a traditional support group, but I know from friends who have experienced other traumas that they can be extraordinarily healing and uplifting. After the loss of her baby, Brianna Turpin and her husband found a local support group comprised of other parents who had lost children. To be in a setting with others to whom they didn't have to explain or excuse their feelings was a massive comfort, Turpin expressed: To know they were not alone, to be with others who truly understood firsthand what they were going through, to find resources. Renowned author, therapist, and Holocaust survivor Edith Eger asserts that there is healing power in telling our truth in the safe presence of others. In her book *The Gift*, she says, "Support groups and twelve-step programs can be a wonderful place to share your truth—and learn from others who are doing the same. Find a local or online meeting where you will be in the company of people who can relate to and empathize with your experience. Attend at least three meetings before you decide whether or not it's for you."[6]

I did have the awesome experience of attending a healing circle organized by one of my closest friends, Belle, the week after the mudslide. Belle assembled a group of my friends and family members and brought in a kundalini yoga teacher and a spiritual healer who led us in rituals where we all, myself included, could cry, be raw, share, and feel that sense of community, to feel like we were all being held by each other.

FOR YOU:

As Eger suggests, find a local or online support group through word of mouth; a referral from a doctor, counselor, or therapist; or by conducting a search online. Consider her directive to attend at least three times before deciding whether it is something you want to continue with or not.

Who is it right for? Wrong for?

Although support groups can be a wonderful way to connect with others who have the life experience to provide empathy and understanding in a way that most of the rest of the population can't, for individuals who are more energy sensitive, I imagine there's the possibility of feeling overwhelmed by the feelings of the group. Sometimes we need time and space, alone time, and one-on-one attention to heal an aspect of our experience, and then perhaps the timing is ripe for the sense of community and connectedness to play its role as the powerful healer. For others, group therapy is a cost-effective way to share, connect with others, and feel validated and supported. It can also be a forum for learning new coping strategies and self-care techniques. Group therapy can also be a way to not feel so alone in the wake of trauma.[7]

TRADITIONAL TALK THERAPY

There are so many styles and different approaches to talk therapy, including more directive styles and more client-led styles. I gravitate to the less rigid, more spiritual, and energetically inclined therapists. Although I find value in honoring and exploring the past, I prefer to focus more on the present rather than participate in traditional psychotherapy heavily focused on the past.

We can all develop certain "adaptive" behaviors and beliefs helpful in navigating and surviving certain situations and relationships in our past. When we bring them forward into the present, they can become "maladaptive" and hold us back or even cause us harm unless we release them. Having a therapist's help to identify and release old patterns and behaviors that no longer serve us is supremely helpful. Alyson Bostwick of Santa Barbara City College, with more than twenty-five years of experience in family systems therapy, shares that trauma in the family can be played out by all of the family members. For example, we might be the identified "healer/fixer/helper" in our family of origin. We did not choose this role but played it to fit in with and survive the (often dysfunctional) family pattern. That role helped our family and helped us exist within it, yet we might grow up and always be drawn to partners who need us to constantly be healing/fixing/helping them. We need to unlearn these unhealthy patterns so that we can have happy, fulfilling relationships, and therapy can help with that.

There is also such value in being seen and heard and having another person be completely present with you. Unfortunately, in everyday life, so many of us are in constant motion and overstimulated and are therefore unable to be present with ourselves, let alone each other. Having a therapist we trust, with whom we can be vulnerable, can allow us to feel truly seen and also be led to the answers we all hold within us for our healing.

Sometimes we think we are the only ones to have such "awful" thoughts or to have done or had done to us such "terrible" things. We feel so alone in our human fallibility and in our suffering. This isolation can be heightened after a trauma. We can find it more difficult to be with people who have no way to understand and relate to what we have been through. Having a good therapist listen, guide, and reframe our personal horrors as acceptable, understandable, and integratable allows us to accept ourselves and the choices we have made and all that we have experienced. It can also offer solace, comfort, and a moment of recognition for our strength and resilience during and after traumatic events.

The people in our lives, our family and friends, can be unsure how to help and support us in the wake of a traumatic event. Their instinct might be to normalize and "get back to life as usual" either as a way of dealing with their own discomfort and fear or as a way to propel us back to "safety." Therapy can shine a light on the fact that these responses, even if they arise from a place of intending to help, can stymie and cause us to repress our healing. We need to work through and process our feelings honestly. A therapist can provide the support and mirroring we are missing in our daily lives.

Bostwick emphasizes the importance of helping her clients change the narrative around trauma, from one of being the victim to being the survivor and placing the blame where the blame belongs. This is particularly true for people who have experienced sexual assault, changing the narrative from "I'm damaged goods" or "I did something to deserve it" to "There's nothing wrong with me that made this happen. There is something very wrong with that person, and I was in the wrong place at the wrong time. I didn't deserve that." Bostwick shares that holding on to the victim mentality can be a crutch for people because it helps us to feel that we have some sort of control, in that if we did something to deserve it, we can change that behavior, when ultimately, we don't have any control. None of us does. Control is an illusion.

I have been going to therapy since I was old enough to get myself to a therapist. As a first-year student at Princeton, I started going to the counseling center, and I have almost always had a therapist in my life since then.

After my second child, India, was born a few months after the mudslide, I found myself sitting on Jenn Paul's couch. Paul was recommended to me as a great postpartum therapist. I originally sought her out to talk about hormonal and life changes following baby number two and then threw in, "By the way, I endured this massive trauma a year ago, but I've been dealing with it!" Basically, "Help me, please."

Paul was warm and friendly and felt familiar. We are about the same age and have kids who had overlapped at the same preschool. Her office was decorated with cheerful prints and pillows, she always had tea and snacks there, and the whir of the air purifier muffled the sounds. I knew her kids had gone to the same preschool my son attended, but because she is very traditional in her strict boundaries and ethics, she rarely talked about herself. She really helped me initially identify that what I had been through was traumatic. I was very much in denial and ready for "life to just go back to normal." She helped me slow down and honor what I had been through so I could begin to process the trauma, to grieve, and to alchemize the fear that still gripped me in a safe, nonjudgmental environment. Therapy with her led to other healing avenues and also allowed me to forgive myself for surviving, for continuing to feel fear, and for being human.

FOR YOU:

The relationship you have with your therapist is incredibly intimate. Ideally in therapy you are sharing and exploring parts and facets of yourself that you might not have had the opportunity to ever look at before. You have the opportunity to try out new behaviors, and you are able to be supremely vulnerable for therapy to be most effective. Because of all of this, working with someone you trust and you like is of paramount importance. Sadly, there are a lot of ill-equipped, ineffective, and in some cases even harmful therapists out there, so be sure to work with someone credentialed (who has the appropriate degree and training). Even better is a therapist recommended by someone you trust.

That being said, trust your gut, interview several therapists, and don't be afraid not to work with someone recommended by family or friends. Bostwick points out that there could be negative transference, meaning that the therapist might remind you of a relative or teacher you have a tricky relationship with, which will cause a negative association, so don't pick that person. Think about what qualities you want in your therapist before you start interviewing, and pick someone you feel you can open up with. Entering therapy is courageous because you have to be vulnerable. As Bostwick says, "Courage is not the absence of fear, but rather the decision that something is more important than fear."

Most insurance companies will cover at least a certain number of therapy sessions. A lot of therapists will work on a sliding scale, and some will even offer pro bono sessions. Working with a licensed social worker can be another option. Additionally, local community clinics can offer low-cost, or even free, counseling services with psychology students who are supervised by licensed therapists. Given the state of technology, therapy can even be conducted over Zoom if you can't find someone ideal to work with nearby.

Who is it right for? Wrong for?

Everyone can benefit from therapy. Everyone! As I mentioned earlier, for therapy to be effective and beneficial, it is critical to find someone you trust and feel comfortable with.

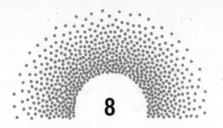

8

Into the Great Wide Open!

How to Heal Yourself with Mystical Therapies

Mystical therapies touch upon multiple dimensions of healing: body, mind, heart, and spirit. They connect to unseen worlds and energies and draw upon ancient and time-tested practices and belief systems that might, for some of you, fall outside your current ideas of what's real or possible.

Miracles happen every day. These modalities work. Trust, openness, and curiosity are required. Although some of these practices have a growing base of scientific support (e.g., meditation, breathwork), others are founded in mystical wisdom passed down for centuries. Because of the nature of many of these practices and their ability to heal without the use of pharmaceuticals and medical devices, these studies lack funding and prioritization, given that the majority of scientific studies are conducted and paid for by the pharmaceutical industry.[1] Be prepared for experiences with mystical healers to surprise and amaze you.

BREATHWORK

Breathwork helps release trauma. Often, we tend to hold our breath while experiencing a traumatic event. Patterned and conscious breathing helps to regulate the nervous system and tap into altered states of consciousness, ultimately shifting our internal landscape. Breathwork is a highly effective practice for moving through trauma and has been used for centuries for healing and spiritual purposes; in fact, the Latin word for "breath" is the same as for "spirit." Author and psychiatrist James Gordon, known for researching and promoting the mind-body connection, teaches soft-belly breathing (breathing in through your nose and out of your mouth while keeping the belly soft) as part of his trauma rehabilitation practice. He shares, "When you breathe slowly and deeply you stimulate the vagus nerve; it quiets the fight-or-flight response, decreases fear and anger, mobilizes self-awareness and capacity for judgment and compassion. It's an antidote right there to fight or flight and to some of the more disturbing effects of trauma."

Holotropic breathwork was created in the 1970s by Stanislav Grof and his wife, Christina Grof. Stanislov Grof is the inventor of transpersonal psychology, a pioneer of lysergic acid diethylamide (LSD) therapy, and a leading expert on non-ordinary states of consciousness. He and his wife developed holotropic breathwork as a way to access the non-ordinary states of consciousness achieved by using LSD, with which Grof had had incredible success in his practice before it became illegal. "Holotropic" comes from the Greek *holus*, which means "whole," and *trepin,* which translates to "progressing toward something," was the most effective legal way they found to induce this state.[2]

In an interview with Dave Asprey of Bulletproof Coffee, Grof explains, "The Holotropic state creates a situation where contents in your unconscious that have a strong emotional charge, close enough to the threshold of consciousness, emerge for processing. It is not up to me (the therapist) to decide what's important. It's basically a process of self-healing." The belief that the body and mind have the innate wisdom to know how to heal is integral to many of these modalities. The modalities that foster and promote our natural flow toward wholeness, health, and harmony are most appealing to me. In repeating our mantra in our wellness retreat business, my sister and I constantly reiterate, "You are your own best guide." There are no gurus; you are the guru of YOU. Grof's perspective on symptoms that manifest after a trauma is that they are an opportunity: "Something is halfway out and is presenting as a call to be fully expelled." The breathwork helps to release the traumatic imprint. Symptoms are merely a tool for discovery.

During holotropic breathwork, we decrease the amount of oxygen and blood in the brain, especially to the areas of the brain that rule visual processing, body sensory information, memory, the experience of time, and the sense of self. The amount of carbon dioxide in the brain and body is also elevated, all of which can lead to powerful hallucinations, otherwise known as visual and introspective experiences, and a general feeling of being in a "waking dream state."[3] This was the practice I dove into with Blake Spencer of Breath of Blake.

I met Blake in a bar. She had just moved to Santa Barbara to deepen her study of trauma therapy (there are no coincidences) and was working at my favorite wine bar, site of my astrology class's postclass hangouts. To practice astrology, we had been studying the charts of everyone who worked there. Blake came by our table, explaining that the owner had sent her over because she was interested in astrology. And the rest is history. We exchanged information, and a few months later it felt like the right time to introduce a new healing therapist and modality to my world.

Blake arrived at my house carrying a colorful woven basket brimming with all sorts of mystical and healing delights: tarot card decks, essential oils, smudging tools, music. We chatted for a while, and she explained what would happen. I would lie down, preferably on the floor, with nothing beneath my head. She would lead me through a series of breaths, all in and out of my mouth, and then act as a guide for me during whatever happened. She explained that my hands might tense up and involuntarily form into claws (they would relax again), I might get cold or hot, and/or I might cry. And so we began.

The initial guided breathing was pretty uncomfortable, and Blake assured me that this "working" part of the practice was almost complete. The breathwork involves an open-mouthed, two-part breath, breathing first into the belly and then into the chest, with a quick exhale. I stuck with it and then began to feel my legs, arms, feet, and hands tingling and vibrating, not uncomfortably. When I shared that my head hurt, Blake said that this was my mind needing to get out of the way, and to keep breathing. And then I had waves of emotion. I was sobbing. The odd thing is, I can't remember exactly what was going through my mind and body, but I know it was releasing some of the grief, fear, and anger I had been storing. And then, as Blake guided me onto a soft "cloud," my body sensations shifted. I was resting my hands on my belly, and I felt something rise up out of my belly into my hand. If you've ever been pregnant, you'll know the feeling of the baby kicking really hard outward, and I was definitely NOT pregnant.

I told Blake I wasn't ready for the "cloud" and described the sensation I was feeling. She asked me what color this sensation was. "Orange," I said.

And I was crying again. "It's the color of the sky the night of the mudslide. The sky was lit up a bizarre orange because of a major gas explosion. That color represented destruction and devastation, and yet I am so grateful to it because without it I wouldn't have been able to see the mudslide. I feel like it saved my and my family's lives." I sobbed and breathed and thanked it. And I felt it go.

Then, Blake lowered me onto the "cloud," and I came back to this world. Wow.

I had no idea how powerful, intense, and effective this session with her was going to be. As I integrated for the few days following, I definitely felt like my head was still in the clouds, but I felt more at peace.

These breathwork sessions are not always so intense. My last session with Blake was more peaceful and euphoric. Although I was excited about this new portal I had discovered, I had a bit of reluctance about continuing with it because I had had such a visceral response. When a friend reached out about a year later inviting me to a session with her breathwork teacher, Gwen Dittmar, I felt like it was an invitation to go deeper and peel back another layer.

Before we started, I told Dittmar about that sensation I'd had in my stomach and that it had felt like an alien rising up and out. She shared that sometimes other entities can invade our bodies and that if it were to happen again, I should ask who/what they were and ask them to leave. So that's how I kicked off that session. I was rather nervous that I had an unwelcome energy living in my belly I was going to have to confront. But this time, although my body got tingly, I felt extreme pressure in my thighs, I had the sensation of being a tube of toothpaste being squeezed, my hands became clawlike, my arms flung out involuntarily, and my mouth contorted a bit, no alien rose up out of my stomach.

In fact, I had this clear knowing that I had been a healer for many lifetimes, that some of the women in the breathwork circle and in my life right now had been my healing sisters in past lives, and that my connection to the orange fire I had seen in the breathwork session with Blake wasn't just about the color the sky was the night of the mudslide. No, the color provoked a knowing in me that I had used fire in mystical, magical rituals lifetimes ago and that also my fear of fire was because I had been burned for my healing abilities (deemed witchcraft at the time). I can't explain exactly how I just *knew* all of this, but I did. The knowing was infused with such calm and understanding of so much, but mostly about who I am and that I am safe in this lifetime to pursue the role of seeker and healer. I will not be killed for it in this lifetime. That was the past.

And then the session was over, and I was flooded with such a serene sense of peace and as if there were infinitely more space within myself. The other women in the session with me all had profound experiences as well. There were a lot of tears of relief, gratitude, and a sense of humility, love, and connection from the group. Sharing with each other afterward, Dittmar explains, helps us integrate and "come back down" to three-dimensional reality. Talking about your experience with the group allows that experience to be brought into your body and your life. It allows for integration, context, clarity, and even the formation of new neural pathways. Closing the session with sharing makes the experience intentional and helps with grounding. If you're having a hard time grounding (you're "floating," spacy, or have a headache) and you don't have issues with alcohol, having a little bit of alcohol can help bring your energy back down into your body, too.

• •

FOR YOU:

There are a lot of books and online tools for doing holotropic breathwork on your own. After my experiences, I would recommend having a guide or practitioner there with you at least the first time you explore this powerful kind of breathwork. Particularly when you are seeking to heal trauma, look for an experienced practitioner, perhaps one who has some sort of trauma-informed background or credential. Dittmar has her master's degree in spiritual psychology and can be reached at her website, gwendittmar.com. She works on a sliding scale and has numerous free videos on her site. She recommends a one-on-one session if at all possible, to move more energy faster while also integrating it. If you start with her videos, begin with the shorter ones (three minutes) and build toward the longer ones as a way of getting acquainted with the practice, your body, and your bodily sensations. Sometimes with trauma we can become dissociated from our bodily sensations as indicators for what and how we're feeling. For example, when I am anxious or retriggered, I tend to feel it in my stomach as an ache, nausea, and so forth. And then I notice that my stomach begins to gurgle in a way that isn't painful, but it is a sign that the energy there is releasing and moving. Blake is in the master's program for trauma therapy at Pacifica and offers sessions over the phone or via Zoom; her website is breathofblake.com.

Another straightforward breathing exercise that can be done anytime, anywhere, and by anyone is simple nasal breathing. As James Nestor outlines in his book *Breath*, "The perfect breath is this: Breathe in for about 5.5 seconds, then exhale for 5.5 seconds. That's 5.5 breaths a minute for a total of about 5.5 liters of air."[4] Nestor reminds us that we don't need apps or gadgets, Wi-Fi, or headgear to practice a calming technique our ancestors have been practicing for centuries. Again, our natural state is one of balance, and our bodies and environment often hold the remedy.

Who is it right for? Wrong for?

Anyone can benefit from holotropic breathwork, and to me it felt like six months of therapy in one session in terms of the magnitude of clearing and healing. The amazing thing I have found, with breathwork personally and in my research, is that whatever needs to and wants to present and come up to be cleared naturally manifests, so no guidance is necessary from the participant or the practitioner in this way. Because it is so powerful, it is important to select an experienced practitioner with a trauma-informed background. Discuss your medical background with your practitioner if you've experienced any unusual symptoms recently. Family histories of manic depression, psychosis, or extremely high or low blood pressure might be indicators that holotropic breathwork might not be safe for you. With any kind of intense breathwork, there is a possibility of passing out, so be sure to practice any deep focused breathing exercises while lying down and never in water.

MEDITATION

Meditation is a practice of quieting the mind and, ideally, accessing other brain wave states. Most of us are often in a beta brain wave state, associated with intellectual thinking, problem solving, and alertness. The goal of meditation is to transition your brain from beta into an alpha or even a theta brain wave state. Alpha, theta, and gamma brain waves are states in which relaxation, creativity, and healing can take place. The overthinking, worrying, vigilant brain state is transcended, and according to bestselling author, researcher, and meditation teacher Joe Dispenza, in the alpha brain wave state, we sense or enter the quantum field. According to Dispenza, the quantum field "is an invisible field of energy and information—or you could say a field of intelligence or consciousness—that exists beyond space and time." In the quantum field, there is no separation; we become awareness and consciousness, and we are in a unified and coherent state. With the analytical mind subdued, coherence exists between the brain and the heart, allowing feelings of ecstasy, instantaneous healing, and manifestation. It can take some practice, so don't be discouraged if you don't reach an ecstatic state your first time!

There are all kinds of meditation; practices in which you are seated with your eyes closed are most common. Usually there is a focus on the breath. Michael Beckwith, founder of the Agape church, a frequent guest on Oprah Winfrey's *Super Soul*, and meditation teacher, says the breath helps keep us present because you can't be breathing in the past and you can't be breathing in the future. Sometimes using a mantra (a short, repeated phrase) can be helpful. Bestselling author and coach Gabby Bernstein describes meditation as a way to "transcend the energy of this world and step into a place of love. Meditation becomes a pathway to the light. . . . The pathway to alignment with the Universe begins with the stillness found in meditation. This is a stillness so deep that you leave the world of perception behind and step into the power of your light."[5]

I learned to meditate more than ten years ago in Venice, California. I attended a free information session in Christian Bevacqua's Venice Beach bungalow. Bevacqua is personable and a lookalike for the actor Jason Schwartzman. He has a compelling backstory: He had graduated from a high-pressure Ivy League school, gone to work on Wall Street, was miserable, had a nervous breakdown, found meditation, quit his job, became a meditation teacher, and moved to Venice Beach. After some internal resistance ("I can't sit still that long! My mind is too busy! Sounds awful"), I signed up along with Lucy and my then boyfriend. Although the beginning was a bit rocky in terms of wandering thoughts, judging myself over doing it "right," and finding and making the time to do it, the incredible calming and euphoric effects soon outweighed my resistance. One thing I loved that Bevacqua helped me with was letting go of attempting to analyze the thoughts and feelings that did come up on their way out, which he likened to the bubbles in a carbonated beverage rising to the surface and then gently releasing. He said, "Think of meditation as if you are taking the trash out. You don't open up your trash and rummage through it before you toss it out, do you?"

Meditation has been one of the best tools I have ever found and has documented positive effects on treating PTSD. I've also witnessed the dramatic and positive effect it has had on other people in my life.[6] The type of meditation I learned from Bevacqua is called transcendental meditation, or Vedic meditation, made famous by the Beatles and David Lynch. One of the more structured practices, it requires a specific training in which each person is given a divine and unique mantra, and meditation is meant to be done for twenty minutes in the morning and twenty minutes in the afternoon/evening. I kept up my rigorous practice of meditating twenty minutes in the morning and twenty minutes in the afternoon/evening for years. As time has gone by, and I have been exposed to other inspiring meditations and meditation teachers, my practice has morphed into a more mom-friendly approach, often requiring less time, and yet a sort of muscle memory existed after I knew how to drop into that healing state; it is easier and quicker to access, and the results are just as palpable.

After the mudslide, I forced myself to meditate even when the horrible images and sounds would force their way in. I believed, as Bevacqua had said many years ago, these images and sounds were bubbling up to be released. My meditation also kept me more balanced, grounded, and hopeful.

Following my meditation in the morning and then again before bed, I would journal as a way to get the heavier and darker thoughts and words out of my head. Also, I did it to record the good things happening for me and my family, to remember and be grateful for the kindnesses shown to us by loved ones and strangers. It was also good to have these gratitude "letters" to look back on when I found myself in darker moments.

• •

FOR YOU:

A great place to start is free guided meditations. Some teachers I love who have different styles and tones are Beckwith, Bernstein, Dispenza, Tara Brach, and Deepak Chopra. They offer free guided meditations on their websites, so explore them all and select the one with whom you resonate.

Here's an easy meditation to start:

- Sit quietly and comfortably, either with your feet on the floor or in a comfortable cross-legged position.

- Close your eyes and begin to deepen your breathing.

- Breathe in through your nose slowly for four to five counts and then exhale through your nose slowly for four to five counts.

- Using the Sanskrit (ancient Indian language) mantra "so hum," which translates to "I am that," with "that" referring to all that is, begin to repeat the mantra to yourself in sync with your breath. Say to yourself "so" on the inhale and "hum" on the exhale.

- Continue for up to twenty minutes. Three minutes is a good place to start, and then build to seven, twelve, and finally twenty minutes. If you lose track of the mantra, no worries.

Who is it right for? Wrong for?

There isn't a living being who couldn't benefit from meditation! It is safe for all ages and is even being offered in some preschools and schools. Mallika Chopra, daughter of Deepak Chopra, has authored several books (*Just Breathe, Just Be You,* and *Just Feel*) on teaching kids to meditate. She speaks of the "privilege of practices" she experienced growing up meditating with her father. I love this idea of giving our children this sort of privilege.

JOURNALING

I have kept a journal for most of my adult life. Journaling can be a therapeutic tool anytime and can help to lessen the effects of trauma while also increasing positive growth from a traumatic event. This is especially true if the focus on the journaling is positive.[7] For me it is a way to externally process what is going on both inside and outside of me. Putting feelings and thoughts on the page helps free up space and energy in my brain and body. I find that writing them down helps me to organize and make sense of my experiences. It also frees me from the sometimes incessant chatter and loops I can get stuck in from time to time.

In my interview with trauma survivor Norma Bastidas, she shared that she journals compulsively as a form of "emotional literacy. Journaling helps me understand my emotions and where they came from, and then it is easier to manage them." She also relies on journaling as a way to manage and keep track of her history. She shared, "I can get confused. The stories can become conflicting, and it is the best way to keep me honest."

Dani Shapiro, author of the bestselling memoir *Inheritance*, relied heavily on writing to move through her trauma. When she discovered through a mail-in DNA test done on a whim that her father was actually not her biological father, she set out on a mission to uncover her true identity, all the while wrestling with overwhelming feelings and sensations of betrayal, groundlessness, and shock. Although her experience didn't feel like "categorizable" trauma, this almost made it harder. She shared, "I am the trauma. My body, the face that looks back at me in the mirror, that is the trauma, and it's so diffuse. How do I go about trying to address this? It's not around an event. It's me."

Shapiro had the opportunity to consult and work with Bessel van der Kolk, one of the world's foremost trauma experts. He writes that those who recover "well" from trauma often have found a way to make meaning out of their trauma. Additionally, adding an element of helping others, giving the trauma a purpose, often allows for a smoother recovery. Shapiro realized that in writing *Inheritance* and in starting a podcast called "Family Secrets" about sharing secrets festering in so many families, she was subconsciously fulfilling this purposeful healing. Having the ostensible purpose of supporting hundreds of thousands of people making discoveries about their genetics helped her metabolize her own shocking discovery.

For me, journaling has a twofold benefit: It helps me understand events that have happened in the past and also helps me manifest the present and future I desire. I find that journaling after meditation allows me greater access to my feelings and provides space for deeper thoughts and emotions to emerge.

The Morning Meeting and Manifesting

In recent years, I have started writing every morning as part of a morning meeting with myself, part of my daily practice. Early in my day, ideally before my kids are awake or after they are at school, I sit quietly with an inspirational book (some favorites are *The Collected Works of Florence Scovel Shinn*; *Living in the Light* by Shakti Gawain; *Ask and It Is Given* by Esther and Jerry Hicks; and *Oneness* by Rasha) and my journal. Pick a blank journal that feels inspiring and good to you; I like ones with birds, butterflies, or bright colors and metallics. I read a few pages of whichever spiritual book I am working my way through, igniting inspiration before I begin to write. As soon as I have the inspired feeling, I open my journal and write.

My writing in these morning meetings takes the form of a letter to myself, any angels and guides, and God, but you can address yours to any higher power, the universe, any spirit, or even your higher self. My letters are grateful, and almost always in the present tense, for feelings, relationships, gifts, and lessons I have received. I also write with appreciation for things I desire that I have yet to receive, but I write in a way in which I already have them. For example, if I desired a new house, I would write, "Thank you for my most perfect home, which is safe, beautiful, and inspiring in the ideal location for the perfect price under grace." You can get more specific with the details (add "which has a luscious backyard," or "with three or more bedrooms," etc.). Writing it as if you already have it puts you in the energetic frequency and vibration of having it, which then attracts it into your life.

Often, we think we are asking for what we want, and we don't understand why we aren't attracting and manifesting our desires. Most of us are asking incorrectly. We are coming from a place of "not having" and lack, which then simply amplifies that energy and pulls more of it into our experience. For example, by writing, "I want a house that I love!" or "I don't want to feel depressed," we are focusing on what is missing, the lack. The lack of a house, the lack of feeling good and happy. Reframing our statements to focus on what we desire as if we already have it is critical. Instead of "I don't want to feel depressed," you would write, "Thank you for the joy and happiness I feel within me and all around me under grace." It is important to add "under grace" because we want to manifest our desires in as easy and gracious a way as possible.

After I have written down all of my desires, including robust and vibrant health for myself, my family, and my community; divinely awesome opportunities; increased abundance under grace; and helping others with ease and grace, I sign off: "For all of this and more and magic, I thank you, and now I release these words to the law, truth, and power of the universe, and it is done. Amen, and I love you." When I am finished writing, I read my words aloud. I have noticed significant and powerful results in manifesting my desires because of this morning meeting practice. It sets my energy and my intentions for the day and for my life. I have manifested desired work outcomes, financial rewards almost to the exact dollar, homes, and happier personal environments through this practice.

I recommend starting with a smaller desire in which there isn't an intense charge (desire) as a way to practice. After these smaller things start manifesting, you will feel reinforced and have greater belief in the science of it all. Because it is science—like attracts like, and all beings and things and situations emit an energetic frequency—the best and most efficient way to attract what you desire is to be it/feel it/emit that frequency. It takes commitment, but I think of this as one of my most important commitments because it is a commitment to myself, God, and creating a life that I love that spreads love! What is more important than that?

Freewriting

Another exercise I like to do is asking the highest version of myself a question and just allowing stream-of-consciousness writing as a response. I don't edit myself or worry about spelling or grammar. It is amazing how we already hold the answers to so many questions we ask, and if we took more time to quiet ourselves and really listen, we would be so much happier! It has been said that prayer is us talking to God, and intuition is God answering us. Often, we are too busy, distracted, or focused on controlling our lives to hear the answers to our prayers coming to us through our intuition. There is no space for our intuition to come through.

Bernstein also finds that through meditation and journaling, she is able to connect with her guides. She defines "guides" as angels or beings with higher consciousness. One way she receives divine guidance is through this connection. After asking her guides for support and/or direction, she meditates and then journals: "I let my pen flow, and don't edit. Write down whatever comes forth, even if it seems mundane or weird at first. Have faith in the process, and allow it to unfold in whatever way it does."[8] If you want to take this exercise a step further, you can write the question with your dominant hand and then switch hands and write the answer with your nondominant hand. Research shows that nondominant handwriting allows for us to access our right brain more easily. The right hemisphere of the brain is responsible for our emotions, intuition, and creativity.

Gratitude journaling

Although my morning meeting journaling is full of gratitude, you can journal this way at any time as a way of reminding yourself of and recording all you are grateful for. This is a great exercise any time of day, but especially before bed because you are imprinting feeling good and grateful on your brain right before sleep. You can write, "I am grateful for coffee, I am grateful for my children, I am grateful for these cozy pajamas, I am grateful for air conditioning, I am grateful for my health, I am grateful for good books." You get the idea: anything and everything you are grateful for. There is a saying that what we appreciate appreciates, so appreciate, appreciate, appreciate. In general, gratitude raises your vibration.

....

FOR YOU:

Get yourself a journal that works for you—you like the look of it, size of it, lined pages or plain, spiral or bound, or whatever suits you. Start small, and commit to writing for a few minutes each day. Build from there.

Who is it right for? Wrong for?
Everyone can benefit from journaling.

SHAMANISM

For our purposes, a shaman has mastered stepping into heightened states of consciousness in order to be a healing force; from the space between dimensions, this person can connect with the power of spirit and channel its energies toward healing. Shamanic beliefs and practices have existed all over the world for most of human history. The word *shaman* means "one who knows," according to Shaman Durek. He goes on to explain in his book *Spirit Hacking*, shamans "act as ambassadors between the physical world and the spiritual world. Shamans utilize a vast array of tools and techniques to communicate with spirits, and ancestors and elements, and all sorts of unseen energies, entities, and intelligences in service to the health of everyone." The distance between what's proven to heal through double-blind studies and the power of shamanic healing might not be as great as you imagine.

In my hometown of Santa Barbara, for example, we have David Cumes, a practicing medical doctor (urologist) and former Stanford University faculty member who is also a *sangoma* (African shaman). I asked Cumes how he bridges these two worlds in his practice. He said they really complement each other because Western medicine is moving toward acceptance of the mind/body connection. Shamanism, he explains, is medicine not localized in space or time. In his African lineage, shamanism allows for ancestors or guides to provide helpful healing information.

I asked Durek to further illuminate some of the ideas about trauma he expounds in his book. He explains that trauma is the pressure that creates the diamond; trauma is the portal to trapped energy not properly released from the physical or emotional body. A traumatic event is an invitation to recognize and get out of the loop keeping you stuck. He shares a poetic visual of a flowering plant that has broken through cement: The flower and all of its growth and cellular regeneration beneath the cement in the earth is akin to what is happening in our bodies and souls when we address, process, and transmute trauma. The cement is all the crap we layer onto the event— shame, judgment, anger, feelings of victimization, and pain—and if we can move through those feelings, the beautiful, radiant flower emerges with a vast network of roots supporting it in the earth. As above, so below.

One of Durek's mantras is "I breathe in darkness and exhale the light." If you don't breathe in the darkness, you'll never heal from your trauma. Acceptance of the totality of trauma is a key component to healing, according to Durek. "Human suffering is due to our nature to create duality; this is bad, or this is good," he explains.

In my struggle to fully grasp this concept, I asked about my experience being molested at the age of seven by a man in his seventies. It was hard for me to fully accept this experience, even more than thirty years later. Durek encouraged me to accept all aspects of the event, then explained that this man had spiritually blessed me through that event. What things had been revealed to me through that experience that I wouldn't have otherwise known? How had that experience been a catalyst for my greatest personal growth? During this conversation, I felt a sense of weighty calmness. Instead of becoming triggered and constricted, I felt as if some locked door had been opened. Out gracefully tumbled a deep breath, and with it, understanding. For me, this understanding came because perhaps enough time had passed, because Durek helped me find this release, or a combination of both.

Therein lies the reframe as well. Through that terrible experience of being molested, I learned to rely on my intuition. I was an old soul who understood in some ways better than the adults around her how to nurture and care for myself. I learned self-reliance, which started me on this path of healing and exploration of what lies beneath the veil and under the surface. Durek says, "Healing occurs when we accept reality as it is, and when we acknowledge that everything happens for the greater good of our being—that our trauma is leading us somewhere. . . . But we will never find out where our suffering is meant to lead us if we don't accept that it happened, and that it happened for our benefit."[9] Take your time, and be gentle and kind with yourself if you find the acceptance a struggle. It took me years and also the right guides, teachers, and a myriad of different therapies to find acceptance.

I happened to find Tim Frank, the shaman I saw after the mudslide, in the middle of the Arizona desert while on a trip. He strode into the cushy waiting room of the spa where I had set up a session with him. He wore a tight black T-shirt and khaki cargo pants and was older than me. He was tan and sort of handsome (but not in a distracting way). In my white, fluffy robe and squeaky spa shoes, with zero idea of what to expect, I followed him out to the yurt where we would be having our session. We bantered about the state of the world as we walked.

We stepped inside the yurt. It felt like a sauna. Two chairs faced each other; a box of tissues was prominently placed on the side table, within reach. A massage table was draped with batik fabric and had what looked like a rattle fashioned from a gourd perched on top. Did I mention that the yurt was very hot?

He told me to have a seat and proceeded to share a bit about his shamanic lineage. He launched into a soliloquy about narcissism, betrayal by humans, and how humanity needs to beg the land for forgiveness.

I interrupted because this was an expensive session, and I was ready to get to "it," whatever "it" was.

"What if *I* need to forgive the *land*?" I asked.

He paused, but I hadn't thrown him.

"People need the land; the land does not need people," he replied. And we were off.

We sat knee to knee and talked about what had happened the night of the mudslide. I explained how I'd felt a brush with death from which I had emerged with little more than splinters, scratches, and a nasty case of poison oak. I'd felt divinely protected.

Frank gave new meaning to this by educating me about shamanic initiation rites. With a near-death experience, there is an initiation to a deeper level of understanding. In shamanism, a trauma in which we sense our life is about to end is regarded as an initiation to a shift in perspective as to how the universe operates. The "death ceremony" is what we experience when our brain and body and soul finally surrender to knowing that no matter what happens, we are going to be okay. Surviving this kind of trauma is an initiation to surrender and showing up for ourselves rather than seeking and searching for solutions and understanding outside of ourselves.

Frank said I had stepped into a role of inspirational teacher and illuminator for so many others who have experienced trauma. To perform this role well, he said, I would have to apply myself to reining in the naughty dog of my mind, especially when it wanted to wander off into negative pastures (which, at the time, was happening quite often).

Together, we formulated a mantra I was to speak at all times: "All encounters, people, and interactions I approach as DIVINE . . . TRANSFORMATION . . . JOY . . . ABUNDANCE . . . PEACE."

Just then, an owl hooted above us. Frank froze and pointed skyward. "The owl is the symbol of the greatest soul death and rebirth. You have had yours, and now you are coming out the other side. Do you think you survived to be taken out now? No! You have work to do. Your job is to live and live happily, with joy, and to be an inspiration for the world."

After drinking a full bottle of water and engaging in more than an hour of conversation with Frank, I disrobed and laid face down on the table. The shaman then moved about me, chanting in various languages, swatting my body with bird wings and tree branches and massaging my limbs with a tingly balm, all while shouting things like:

"Choose life!"

"Your life is just beginning, Mare!"

"You hold the heart of humanity!"

"Show me the way!"

. . . into my ears.

He inserted acupuncture needles all over my body. Massaging, drumming, chanting, and the aroma of burning herbs almost overwhelmed me as I laid there in a semiconscious state—wanting to take in what was happening, willing myself to go with it and not judge it, and wanting to be open to releasing stagnated fear and trauma, to stepping forward into my light and power and to being empowered to blaze my trail to uplift others.

He had me flip over, cracking my back as I turned (which felt amazing!), and then placed what felt like a hot, heavy bag of cement on my abdomen, which wrapped around my sides. More massaging, more drumming, more chanting into my ears and over my body. And then this frenzy of healing and clearing was done.

I felt like I'd had spiritual surgery. I was so grateful! I donned my white robe and threw my arms around the shaman. He told me not to talk to anyone right away because I'd be an empathic sponge for quite a while after this session. "Go to the waters," he ordered. "Sink to the bottom. And when you are ready," he pointed upward, "you tell God you are ready to be an inspiration and light the way."

In the dusky twilight of the Arizona desert, I found my way back to the spa, dropped my robe, and sank to the bottom of the whirlpool in the women's locker room. As luck would have it, the locker room was deserted. After sinking and floating up for chlorine-laden air several times, I pointed to the heavens and said: *I am ready!*

• •

FOR YOU:

Cumes explained the concept of "energetic pollution" to me. Often, after a trauma or death, there can be residual energy. Clearing this energy helps us move forward freely and with our health. Ancient civilizations knew this; for example, the Zulus would perform ritual energetic cleansings for their warriors when they returned from war. Cumes also warned against keeping weapons or other items used for killing or dark magic in your home as they can hold and emit that energy. For example, your great-great-grandfather's silver revolver he used in the Civil War—maybe you don't want to keep that! That cool tribal mask from New Guinea used in sacrificial rituals—might want to rethink keeping that around!

Although there isn't really a substitute for working in person with a shaman, in his book *Spirit Hacking,* Durek shares two exercises you can do on your own to release trauma. The book is an excellent resource if you want to dive deeper into shamanism.

- Tapping the wrist: As we know by now, the body constricts during trauma and can remain so unless we release it. Tap the inside of your wrist, which is a direct line to the heart, while saying aloud, "Release the constriction and trauma from your body now." (It is important to speak in the third person.) Breathe deeply.

- Clothes are another form of control over our need to feel vulnerable. Get vulnerable and remove all of your clothing.

Lying naked on a bed, say out loud, "I want you to start breathing deeply, and start releasing deep trauma from your body now." Again, speak in the third person.

• • • •

EXERCISE

You might incorporate these exercises into a larger magical ritual by setting aside an hour or two, preferably where you will be undisturbed:

1. Begin by clearing yourself and your space by burning palo santo (this sweet-smelling wood from a South American tree is often used to purify and elevate spaces; buy some online or in a local shop that carries items like this). Leave a window or door open so that the smoke can remove what it needs to from the space and then have a place to exit. You wouldn't bang off your dusty, muddy shoes inside your house, would you? This is the same idea.

2. After your space is cleared, light a candle with intention. Say a prayer or read a poem or piece of writing that feels illuminating. Then, state your intention out loud for what you wish to accomplish with the ritual. For example: "I am creating peace, harmony, love, and abundance in my inner and outer world."

3. It can be an added help to hold weighty crystals in each hand. Crystals amplify and shift energy with the vibrations they emit, which work with our own electromagnetic fields. A few of my favorite crystals are rose quartz (helps open the heart and allow for more love), black tourmaline (to ward off negative energy), citrine (promotes joy, creativity, and abundance), and amethyst (relaxes us and helps us tap into our intuition).

4. After setting up your ceremonial environment, meditate, focusing on your breath in and out. Focus on grounding and releasing what isn't working for you. Let it go! Picture roots

growing from the bottom of your feet (or the base of your pelvis, if you're sitting on the floor) down into the earth and anchoring you by wrapping around a beautiful crystal.

5. Then, imagine pulling that powerful earth energy back up through the ground into your body.

6. As a complement to the earth energy, imagine that you are opening the top of your head to a warm, clarifying, love-filled light. Picture the light flooding your body and the space around your body. Stay with it for a few minutes.

7. When you feel complete after at least three minutes and up to twenty, slowly open your eyes. Take some time to return from your journey inward.

8. Write down all you are releasing and letting go of, and write about all you are healing. Burn the piece of paper you've written on.

9. Bells are a good thing to have on hand; the ringing of bells helps break up stuck and stagnant energy. Ring those bells if you've got 'em! Get up and dance and shake. Imagine you are shaking up and off anything that no longer serves you, and that you are making space for all that you *do* desire.

10. After a good dance party shake-off, mist yourself with some sweet-smelling rose spray (I like Heritage Store's Rosewater).

11. Settle back down and take out your journal to declare all you are grateful for in your life. Write your desires in the present tense *as if they have already manifested.* Feel the emotions achieving these desires will bring: love, acceptance, fulfillment, joy, limitlessness, peace. This primes your body and your mind to be in a state of receptiveness and attraction rather than attempting to create from a place of wanting and lack.

12. When you feel complete with your writing, read it aloud with conviction.

13. End by burning some sweetgrass, which is thought to attract positive energies.

Who is it right for? Wrong for?

Shamanism can draw some of its power from the darker realms such as voodoo. It shouldn't be entered into lightly. In my experience, it is best to explore shamanism from a more grounded place after you've been on your healing journey for a little while. Also, be sure to work with someone recommended with whom you feel safe, and if something doesn't feel right, don't do it. The rituals outlined above are safe to do.

PSYCHOLOGICAL ASTROLOGY

I've always been interested in all aspects of what makes people who they are, including cosmically. I was fortunate that my good friend Jennifer Freed came into my life a few years before the mudslide. In addition to having her PhD in psychology, she is a seasoned and passionate astrologer who has been studying and reading charts for more than forty years.

The first time I met her was to have her read my chart. She was spot on, even if I didn't like some of what she shared with me. I also had the experience of taking one of her astrology classes for six months, which was illuminating and empowering all at once. Although it seems there are certain universal truths to some aspects of astrology, there are also infinite possibilities in terms of how planets and stars and their aspects manifest in a human life experience.

Most people know what their astrological sun sign is; however, there are two other critical aspects to understand about astrology. Your sun sign, meaning where the sun was at the time of your birth, essentially influences your personality. Your moon sign, or where the moon was at the time of your birth, represents deep, non-negotiable emotional needs that are critical for your happiness and flourishing as a human being. The moon can also represent your relationship to your mother. Finally, your rising sign, otherwise known as our ascendant, is the zodiac sign rising on the eastern horizon at the exact time of your birth. Your rising sign represents how you present outwardly to the world. You can think of it as the rising sign being your public persona and your sun sign as being your true nature. When reading horoscopes, always read both your sun and rising sign.

While I was in Freed's astrology class, learning about my moon sign, I noticed that my moon is conjunct (meaning in direct relationship to) Chiron in my chart. Chiron is the planet that represents our deepest spiritual wounds. Astrologer Adam Sommer explains,

> Chiron is the world's first centaur. He carries orphan wisdom, in that his father Saturn galloped off after conception, and his mother Philrya begged to be released when this mutant child was born, so she was turned into a linden tree. Chiron was raised by the wild. The Sun and Moon (Apollo & Artemis) were his surrogate parents. In time, he became the most esteemed teacher in the ancient world. His cave was a hero factory where he trained young gods, demigods, and mortals how to face their destiny. One of these students, Hercules, accidentally shot him with a poison arrow one ill-fated day, and it was a poison that could not be worked with. The finest healer in the world was left in paradox: He could heal others, but not himself. We too are left with a similar paradox. Somewhere, deep inside of all of us, this story is playing out. There is orphan wisdom in there. There is paradoxical medicine as well. There are wild teachings. In the end, Chiron is who helps us with all our traumas. On clear summer nights, you can still see him out there, teaching from the center of our galaxy, bow pulled back, ready for anything.

I became alarmed by my Venus/Chiron conjunction because who wants a wound amplifying one's heart's desires? When I asked Freed about this alignment, she was completely unfazed: "Of course, the wounded healer. You're a healer, I have that too. Any healer worth their snuff has that aspect. Otherwise how could you truly empathize and help anyone else with their healing?"

Once again, this idea that our wounds and traumas bring greater understanding, compassion, and ability to relate to ourselves and others presented itself. Our deepest wounds can become powerful strengths as well as a way to our purest love and sense of being in the world. Sommer provides us some clues as to how to decipher our traumas in our astrological charts:

> Traditionally, trauma is shown as the two 'malefics,' Mars and Saturn, that would be studied as the cause of the trouble. These days, the outer planets that are transiting (currently moving overhead in the cosmos)

have much to say about the trauma we must experience to awaken our Soul. It is Neptune who wakes us up, Uranus who shocks us into a novel perspective, and Pluto who touches us with death and what stirs in the shadows. When they transit (move over) something important in our charts, something like trauma is likely.

These transits are not to be feared because through these experiences, our "souls are awakened," as Sommer so eloquently states.

Each sign has its strengths and its challenges. Again, it is important to consider your whole chart and that each person's chart is unique; however, sometimes generalizations can be made. New moons, which happen every thirty days, are always a good time to reset and actively choose how you would like to grow, but as Freed says, "The best time to address something is when you notice it's interfering with your well-being."

. . . .

FOR YOU:

You can calculate your birth chart for free on numerous online programs. One I like is astrodienst.com. After you know your sun, moon, and rising signs, there are many brilliant astrologers to consult with. Freed's book *Use Your Planets Wisely* breaks down each sign as to how we can best harness our potential as well as pitfalls to be aware of regarding that sign. Sommer's website, holestoheavens.com, is another good resource. Other astrologers I like are Chani Nicolas, Virginia Rosenberg, and Mystic Mamma.

Who is it right for? Wrong for?

Freed explains that astrology can provide a map for navigating your best path forward and even which healing modalities might be most beneficial for you. Remember, there is limitless access to astrologers, and some of them might present information in unhelpful or even harmful ways. Don't be too swayed by any forecasting, particularly if it is ominous. That might be a time to consult one of the astrologers I mention and to remember what Sommer says about a "challenging" transit coming our way: "Work with the fear. To quote Frank Herbert, 'Fear is the mind-killer.' We need imagination instead. To see the transit as an opportunity to create and imagine our way through it. Nothing is more exciting than a once-in-a-lifetime transit. Invite it in fully."

PRAYER

The power of prayer has been used for thousands of years as a means of feeling relief, manifesting desires, and creating a sense of support both spiritually and physically. Praying in community amplifies our individual prayers, some people believe. Gabby Bernstein talks about prayer as a way of surrendering to the guidance all around you; prayer is a way of turning "it" over to the universe and asking for help. She writes in *Super Attractor*, "A prayer reclaims your faith in a higher power and is a humble request to transcend the false, fear-based beliefs of the world and remember the light of who you are."

It is comforting to believe we are not alone and there are forces greater than us, whether we believe in God, the universe, angels, or a higher self, and that when we pray, we are asking for guidance as well as putting ourselves in a state of allowing. Prayer might be thought of as the question and intuition the answer. My conversation with Michael Beckwith, founder of Agape International Spiritual Center, a transdenominational movement and community of thousands of members and millions of live streamers, felt like a divine experience.

Beckwith explained patiently that we must understand what God is:

God is not a man in the sky doling out good for good people and bad for bad people. God is a presence that is never in absence. God is everywhere. The presence and essence of God is love, intelligence, beauty, abundance, all these qualities, and it is everywhere except where it is suppressed by limited perception. If one's perception is limited, then your experience of the presence of God is suppressed and limited. People have a tendency to think superstitiously: *This earthquake happened, this mudslide happened, God must have done this!* Now, those things happen in nature for various reasons. Gravity is happening all the time. Think about the equator: When the equator gets too hot, the way it cools itself is by creating hurricanes and tornadoes; that's how it sweats, the same way our body sweats to cool itself. These things can be explained through nature. . . . From scripture, "God is not a respecter of persons." The presence of God responds to our vibration. Life responds to the nature of our song.

I asked Beckwith to explain why bad things happen to good people. His response was what he calls the Four Windows of Manifestation:

1. Thoughts: We experience what we think about most. As Job said, "What I feared most came upon me." People elicit the Job Effect; what they are afraid of they bring to themselves by law or out of ignorance and limited perception. We experience our thoughts and perceptions whether conscious or unconscious.

2. Learning a Lesson: The universe is progressive. It is always expanding. Let's say someone prays for more health or prosperity in their life; things will be set in motion for that person to grow. And as they are growing, some of the things that are happening may not be labeled as "good." There may be a change in relationship, they may be suffering some losses, many things may happen that could be labeled as "bad" or "terrible," but as time goes on, they realize if that bad thing hadn't happened to me, I wouldn't be where I am today. I wouldn't have learned kindness, compassion, generosity. What looked like something bad from one perception becomes something transformational from another perception. They put themself on a learning curve by inviting something into their life (I want to be healthier, more prosperous). In order to be the person to have those things, you actually have to become that person. You have to grow into that.

3. Blessing: There are people who come to the planet, and part of their agenda in being here is to raise the love ethic of humanity. To foster and bring more compassion and kindness. These individuals may take on certain experiences in order to bring about compassion in a person's life. For example, a woman was stuck; she had a lot of money, but her heart was not open. She gave birth to a little boy who was born mentally challenged. The woman fell in love with the little boy. When the little boy was twelve, he fell into the pool and drowned. That boy, his birth and his death, opened her heart. His life was a gift to open her heart. What looked like a tragedy was also a blessing. There are people who are born who take on debilitating oppression sometimes in order to open the heart of humanity so that we can say, "Never again!" and grow in compassion. The Jewish holocaust, the African holocaust, the Vietnam War holocaust. People come in and sometimes

seemingly terrible things happen, but out of those terrible things, humanity evolves into greater compassion.

4. Collective Consciousness: As long as there is a belief in scarcity, lack, and not enough, someone will be here to experience them. Until they are eradicated from the mental atmosphere, people will experience these states unconsciously because in reality none of these things exist. There is no lack, no scarcity, no limitation in the quantum field. As the Bhagavad Gita says, "If you take abundance from abundance, abundance still remains." We are only experiencing our beliefs. As long as these beliefs exist in the collective consciousness, we can still experience them unconsciously.

This explanation of experiencing states, emotions, and manifestations from the collective helped something click for me. So many religious teachings, spiritual texts, and practices promoting enlightenment speak of this idea of oneness and unity. If someone is suffering halfway around the world, on some level we all experience that, they believe. I could never quite wrap my head around this concept, although my heart was open to it. I couldn't wrap my conscious mind around it because the manifestation of the collective in our own lives is *unconscious*. Until we eradicate these false beliefs of lack, scarcity, and separateness from the collective, we *will* all experience them to various degrees in our own experience, unconsciously, although they will manifest on a conscious level in one way or another. This is true for both desirable and less desirable states. It behooves us all to aspire and work toward eradication of these limiting false beliefs and focus on and amplify more of what is desirable.

To keep yourself and your unconscious clear and in as positive a state as possible, Beckwith recommends no fast food, only limited exposure to mass media, and no low-calorie conversations (no gossip). He refers to a study about mass media that found that if you repeat a lie enough times, people defend it as the truth. This was in Hitler's playbook; the only difference between the truth and a lie is repetition. When I then asked in reference to Hitler if evil exists, Beckwith responded that some people are disconnected from their souls, and they do evil things. Is that person inherently evil? No, that person is ignorant. *Behind every human aberration there lies a spiritual aspiration.* Under the aberrant behavior, an energy is trying to emerge, but it is coming through a personality that is hurt or wounded. Auschwitz survivor, author, and psychologist Edith Eger echoed this by quoting Anne Frank, who, although witnessing people committing atrocities from the window where she remained hidden, said: "I still believe that people are basically good." Eger continues, "We aren't born to hate. We are taught to hate."

I have been a spiritual person since, as a teenager, I went to a camp that emphasized religion. Although I attended a Christian girls' school, church, and Sunday school, which all felt pretty joyless, ironically devoid of spirituality, it wasn't until that summer at camp when I felt the real love and connection to a power greater than what I could perceive with my senses. This sense of "God" or some greater universal force grew for me, and I embraced aspects of myriad religions as I learned about them. These days, I would consider myself spiritual rather than religious. I pray daily, and I palpably felt a presence with me the night of the mudslide that was calming, loving, and there to protect me. I certainly was praying a lot that night, and I felt divinely protected.

Granted, there are countless styles of praying and expressing spirituality. An observation on gospel-style prayer services and gatherings is that they blend many modalities that help heal trauma. There is often movement through dance or expressive bodily gestures; there is singing, which is using one's voice and creating a resonant healing vibration in the body both by emitting sound and by essentially bathing in the sound all around you; there is the power of community; and there is the acknowledgment of some sort of higher, loving power.

After a traumatic event, we can feel isolated and alone, which is why coming together can be healing in and of itself. Beckwith's Agape services are designed to be a vehicle for greater love and peace. The word *agape* is Greek for "unconditional love." Agape was founded as a "local and global trans-denominational spiritual 'center,'" as a way to embrace and celebrate diversity and inclusion. At the heart of the Agape program is this notion that we are "co-creative participants [with a higher power] in this three-dimensional world in which we live." Beckwith shapes and delivers spiritual teachings and philosophies in a modern and accessible way with an aim to help all parishioners live with greater love so they can offer their unique gifts to the world. His sermons pull from sacred texts, including the Gnostic-inspired bible translated from Aramaic, the Bhagavad Gita and *Yoga Sutras of Patanjali*, *Tao Te Ching*, Kabbalah's Zohar, works by the transcendentalists, and more.

In response to how best to approach healing after trauma, Beckwith encourages us to ask empowering questions rather than ones that are disempowering by casting us in the role of victim. Instead of asking, "Why me?," ask the more empowering question, "What is trying to emerge through me as I'm going through this?" "What good is here that I presently cannot see?" "What kind of person do I want to be when this is over?" "If this particular event/circumstance were to last forever, what quality would I have to embrace in order to have peace of mind?" When we ask these questions, our attention goes to that possibility. *You are not a victim; you are in a very intense growth experience.* When you come through this, you will be different. Focus on something different, and you will be empowered.

He shared the story of Clarence Chance, who was wrongfully incarcerated for seventeen years for a crime he didn't commit. While he was in jail, Chance learned to meditate, and he studied. Although he was incarcerated, his soul was not. When he was released, he shared with Beckwith a story about seeing two people in an argument over a fender bender. His comment was, "There are more people imprisoned out here than there are in jail! There are more people imprisoned by their thoughts and emotions than there are in jail." Chance said that going to jail was the best thing that ever happened to him because he wasn't on the streets. He could have done something bad, but he didn't; he "woke up" because jail became a cauldron of transformation for him.

From Beckwith's perspective, meditation is a key tool for healing from trauma. Through meditation, you can be led from reaction to growth. Meditation reframes behavior and thoughts at a higher level. It changes your interior awareness so that you can transform, and transformation doesn't always look or feel good. Just as the caterpillar turns to liquid in the chrysalis before it emerges as a butterfly, sometimes our circumstances or we ourselves "fall apart" before we emerge as butterflies. Beckwith practices and teaches vipassana meditation and says that any meditation practice will be effective as long as it is approached with sincere motivation. What he means by this is that when you are earnest, you practice whether you feel like it or not. His style of meditation, which he has taught for more than forty years, looks like this: Set your intention; embrace your intention with your attention; focus on the breath, which keeps you present (you can't breathe in the past or the future); sit as if someone is about to tell you the greatest secret in the world, so that you are available and receptive to seeing without eyes and hearing without ears. And then move into the space of beginner's mind, as if this is were your first time practicing. Every time.

I asked Beckwith how we might learn to pray "better." He said the way one prays is affected by your perception of God; if you think God is far away from you and has human tendencies, then you are going to try to manipulate God or change God's mind about you and your circumstances. When you realize God is everywhere, you become more conscious that you already have what you are praying for; you are just blocking yourself from having it. You are praying to clean up your own awareness so that the presence, which is always giving and broadcasting its nature, can be expressed through you. You are praying for the realization of your oneness with God. If anything is lacking (health, prosperity, etc.), it is only lacking in appearance because it is all within you.

. . . .

FOR YOU:

Prayer can be practiced by anyone, anywhere, anytime. There are many resources, including live streaming and prerecorded Agape services on Beckwith's Agape website, agapelive.com. His own website, michaelbeckwith.com, and his social media accounts have other resources, including meditation classes and more.

Bernstein's website, gabbybernstein.com, has other inspiration, tools, tips, and classes. She recommends *A Course in Miracles* by the Foundation for Peace.

A quick prayer I love that you can try is, "Thank you for this day, for my breath, my healthy body, love, beauty, and showing up as the greatest expression of love and kindness. How does it get even better than this?"

Who is it right for? Wrong for?

Unfortunately, some of us were raised in less-than-loving religious settings, or for whatever reason have a negative connotation or associations with the concepts of God, religion, and prayer. If your trauma is related to religion, I suggest starting with other healing modalities listed in the book that resonate with you before approaching prayer. Again, the kind of prayer I'm talking about is not affiliated with a specific denomination or religion. I'm talking about *spirituality rather than religion*, meaning believing in yourself, something bigger than yourself, and the power of love and goodness and light. We can all benefit from that.

SOUND HEALING

Everything has a frequency and a vibration. As human beings, we can vibrate at different frequencies, some of which feel calming and euphoric, whereas others might leave us feeling frustrated, confused, or apathetic. The vibrations that different sounds emit affect our own vibrations. Discordant, loud, intense tones can elicit feelings of anger and aggression, and harmonious melodies and tones can be intensely soothing, relaxing, and healing. Jonathan Goldman is an international author, speaker, and teacher of sound healing and harmonics who directs the Sound Healers Association. He explains sound healing as

> the use of sound to create balance and alignment in: the physical body, the energy centers called "chakras," and/or the etheric fields. The sound may be applied by an instrument or by the human voice. Sound Healing is a vibrational therapy and can be understood as being energy medicine. Sound encompasses virtually all aspects of the auditory phenomenon—from music to nature sounds to electronic sounds to vocal sounds. Practitioners who use sound may likewise use anything that falls within this scope; from classical music to drumming and chanting to electronically synthesized sounds to acoustic instruments.[10]

Sound healer and Reiki practitioner Danielle Kunkleman, with whom I personally worked, explained that although we are all unique, one frequency, 432 hertz, creates universal harmony and a trancelike state. A hertz represents the number of sound wave cycles per second. Kunkleman uses crystal bowls that are all tuned to 432 hertz. Different instruments are used at different points during her clients' session, or journey, as she refers to it. She uses chimes to call in an airy and open feeling. She might employ a rattle or drum to help shake up the energy so that what needs to be released can be. She uses silence so that clients can see/feel/be where they are. Then she rings the bowls to tap into the "eternal void," where the healing occurs. She closes her sessions the same way she begins them, with chimes. She states that it is important to close the session like this because leaving people in the trancelike state the bowls can induce can be really disorienting.

My accidental foray into sound healing happened several years ago before I knew anything about it. My sister, Lucy, and I were visiting Joshua Tree in California when we came upon the Integretron, a dome-shaped white building in the middle of nowhere in the desert. We had heard "sound baths" were performed there and were intrigued. We showed up for our appointment, entered through the metal gates, and wondered if anyone was there because it felt deserted, rather like a reception venue after the party. As we approached the dome, an older man came out, introduced himself, and explained he would be our guide while we were there. He relayed the otherworldly history of the property: It was built by George Van Tassel in the 1950s as an "electrostatic generator for the purpose of rejuvenation and time travel." We were shown framed news clippings that lined the walls of the first floor and included photographs of people in beautiful dresses and tuxedos who looked like movie stars. Our guide explained that these "people" were actually extraterrestrials from Venus who had come in an unidentified flying object (UFO) that landed near the property. Van Tassel was known to believe in and work to contact UFOs.

Suspending our doubts and going along with the story, we climbed the stairs to the second floor, the glorious wooden dome. The acoustics were incredible. Lucy and I could hear each other perfectly when one of us whispered on opposite sides of the fifty-five-foot circumference dome. There were yoga mats, blankets, and props arranged in a circle inside the dome. Our guide showed us each to a mat and explained that we were to get comfortable. While we laid there, he would play the twenty quartz singing bowls, each one emitting a different frequency that would "nourish and restore each of our chakras and energy centers." We closed our eyes and soon thereafter forgot where we were because we were transported to a deep, almost meditative or trancelike state. We both shared afterward that we felt waves of joy, relaxation, and peace as the sound waves harmonized our bodies and minds. We were also stunned to discover that what had felt like a pleasant twenty minutes was actually an hour and a half! Whether our guide was actually an alien from Venus or we had been transported to another era, time had been suspended for us for that hour and a half, and we loved our experience.

My recent and more formal sound healing experience with Kunkleman was transcendent and much more focused. We spoke for a while first and shared our dedication to the path of posttraumatic growth and, as Kunkleman so eloquently stated, "for people to know there is another way, especially in a society that capitalizes on pain." We didn't dwell on the traumatic events that had led me to seek deeper healing; we touched upon them, acknowledging how in other forms of therapy the story can become your identity. Talking about and retelling the traumatic events of our lives can be counterproductive to the healing! She related how sound healings had helped her personally and said that we are all sound healers because we all have a voice.

Humming is something all of us can do that has so many healing and helpful benefits. In *The Humming Effect*, Goldman asserts that, with humming, not only can we lower stress and induce an uptick in oxytocin, our body's "feel-good chemical," but also we can enhance our sleep and lower our blood pressure. Humming is a gentle way to ground ourselves back into our bodies by using our voices to emit a healing vibration.

I laid down on a massage table fully clothed, and Kunkleman anointed me with Blue Lotus oil, thought to aid in dispelling negative energy and help open the third eye. She began to lead me in breathing, inhaling a white diamond light and exhaling "soot," anything I needed or wanted to let go. She talked me through several cycles of breath, and I felt my body relax and my stomach gurgle and settle. What followed felt like a lovely reverie, and I can't be entirely sure of the order in which things unfolded, a further testament to how relaxing and healing my experience was. Kunkleman played chimes and walked around my body, calling in my guides and any angels. She guided me to imagine roots growing from me and anchoring me into the earth. She asked me if there was anyone draining my energy, and to picture them and then with love cut the energetic cord between us with a sword made out of selenite, a white crystal known for its cleansing and protective powers.

We filled my body and the space around my body with golden light. She played the crystal bowls, which made me feel euphoric. For those who meditate, it compares to the euphoria that can come during deep meditation. I felt the vibrations and the resonance in my body. She sang a beautiful song about water and letting the water flow around me. She played a recording of something that sounded like a Native American prayer or poem, and although I can't recall the exact words, it felt empowering and settling all at once. And then she played the chimes again and gently brought me back to my body and this three-dimensional reality.

I felt calm after our session. I felt that stagnant energy had been removed from me, leaving me more open to hope and possibility. I felt lighter. I felt like water, a still, calm, clear lake. I felt safer in my body and in my house. I was more patient with my children that evening, and I moved through the following days with a greater optimism. Although we didn't directly work on my specific traumas, we worked on the whole me, the energy I had been carrying, projecting, perpetuating, and guarding against. We gently helped me shed some of the maladaptive frequencies by reminding the whole of me that I *am* whole and that when I am in alignment, this peace and joyful expectation exists. It exists all the time within me and around me, but if I am stuck in a fight-or-flight response or the residue that response leaves behind, anxiety or depression, I can't stop and smell the roses or appreciate their beauty. I'm busy getting ready to fight or flee. My session with Kunkleman was a beautiful reminder that I am not stuck in my traumatic state; I am able to slow down, to recalibrate, and to recognize and resonate with the frequencies of love and beauty. As Kunkleman so eloquently said about her own posttraumatic growth, she stepped into the witness state of being unattached to her story. In her posttraumatic growth state, she is nonreactive and experiences the aliveness of everything once again or maybe even for the first time.

FOR YOU:

Humming is something Kunkleman does to help ground and reset her energy. Humming is available to us all most of the time. She shared one ritual she practices using water combined with sound. While in the shower, hum and imagine that the water is golden and is cleansing you of all the accumulated sticky, mosslike energetic gunk. As you step out of the shower, imagine you are stepping into a new quantum reality with a higher vibration. Kunkleman offers one-on-one sessions both in person or online and has a YouTube channel with prerecorded sound healings and meditations. Her website is foxysage.com.

Be sure to drink a lot of water after your session, and even add some electrolytes. I am an avid water drinker, and yet moving that much energy is a lot of work, and I was definitely a bit dehydrated and nauseated the following day as my body recalibrated. Don't be alarmed by these physical sensations, or even if you feel a bit "stirred up" after a session. I remind myself that these sensations and emotions are signs that my whole self is healing and growing and that although I am a little bit uncomfortable, the transformation is a good thing. It's like growing pains.

Goldman also offers a lot of resources, some of them free, on his website, healingsounds.com, full of articles, books, musical downloads, chakra tuning apps, and more.

Who is it right for? Wrong for?

Sound healing is a gentle approach to healing and can benefit any-one and everyone. It may also be especially good for people in the beginning of their healing journey because it doesn't require active communication from the participant. Regardless of your timing, if you prefer healing methods that don't require you to speak, then this is a good one for you. Sound healing allows for you to be able to be more passive and receive healing. That being said, be gentle with yourself after the healing session and recognize that a lot of work has been done and that your energetic body is integrating, composting, alchemizing, and recalibrating.

PAST LIFE REGRESSION THERAPY

I read Brian Weiss's *Many Lives, Many Masters* years ago, when I was about thirteen years old. I was fascinated by the idea of reincarnation and the no-tion that feelings, sensations, and relationships we have in this lifetime might be tied to past life experiences. While I was writing this book, Weiss's work came up on my radar again, and this time I took the perspective of being curious about how understanding our past lives could help us heal current trauma in this lifetime.

Weiss is a psychotherapist who holds degrees from Columbia and Yale Universities. He stumbled into the world of past life regression therapy while working with a patient, "Catherine," in the 1980s. According to Weiss, past life regression therapy is another method of eliminating fear, which leads to healing. He also emphasizes that your subconscious mind, accessed during the regression, will never give you more than you can handle or lead you to a place of pain and suffering. We are hardwired to heal.

In his books, Weiss gives several examples of how psychological and phys-ical spontaneous healing can result from accessing the memory of a past life in which a trauma occurred. For example, a patient experiencing unex-plained shoulder pain might do a past life regression in which they see that they were stabbed in the shoulder. When they wake from the hypnotic state, the shoulder pain is gone. Or someone with an unexplainable fear of water might do a past life regression and see that they drowned. According to past life regression therapy, this can resolve the fear of water in this lifetime.

I really wanted to work with Weiss, but he is retired, and I was on a hunt to find someone else, having no luck. In my session for sound healing with

Kunkleman, we were talking about all sorts of healing modalities she had experienced, with incredible results, when she asked, "Have you ever tried past life regression therapy? I have the absolute best person." She connected me with past life regression therapist Niki Cozmo, then and there.

Past life regression therapy uses hypnosis as a means of accessing and recovering memories stored in the subconscious. These memories can be from this lifetime, including infancy, or from previous lifetimes. I was excited to explore this possibility because my healing journey kept leading me to more and more clues as to how to understand, accept, and integrate my experience to ultimately thrive.

Cozmo lost her father, mother, and only sibling before the age of thirty. She spent the next few years traveling the world, learning and experiencing as much as she could from as many different schools of thought as possible. She feels that with each death of a family member, she was cosmically catapulted to a new dimension and that she "catalyzed her pain into purpose," launching her healing business after her sister's death. Her experience of navigating these traumas and her grief led her to explore all manner of healing modalities, both as the receiver and the giver. The healing powers of hypnosis and past life regression therapy resonated with her, and she completed intensive training in each. According to Cozmo, science states that energy can neither be created nor destroyed; therefore, the life force, energy, soul, or spirit must be continuous before we are born and after we die. This explains the concept of past lives; although this physical body will expire, the soul goes on, and it has inhabited other bodies in other lifetimes. The memories from all of these previous lifetimes are stored in the subconscious mind, unavailable to us unless we access them through hypnosis. By unlocking our subconscious through hypnosis, we are shown information from previous lifetimes that can help us in this current lifetime.

I asked Cozmo if there is anyone who can't be hypnotized. She claims that everyone is able to be hypnotized, and in all of her years of hypnotherapy and past life regression work, only two clients have not been able to surrender to hypnosis, at first. In both cases, significant traumatic events were uncovered that had led to the creation of such significant defenses so as to prevent access to them.

My session with Cozmo, conducted over Zoom, began with her asking a bit about my history and my hopes for the session. She pointed out that getting fixated on something you want to see doesn't help and can actually deter you from seeing and absorbing what you're being shown. So, she said not to be too attached to an outcome and to go with what came up. She explained the subconscious versus conscious mind and stated that almost 95 percent of our consciousness is subconscious![11] That means that we are only accessing 5 percent of our consciousness consciously. And many "truths" that we hold in our subconscious minds are implanted there between the ages of zero and eight. These "truths" can be something an authority figure said or repeated to us as children that got implanted. Being told repeatedly that broccoli makes you strong or that children should be seen and not heard are examples of how what we are told as children between these ages can register and be recorded as facts, or truths.

Cozmo then explained that the nonverbal part of the session was beginning. She asked me a series of questions and said I should shake my head for "yes" or "no" in order to help her help me. She asked, for example, "With a new group of people, do you feel comfortable initiating conversation?" Yes. "Do you prefer fiction to nonfiction?" That was sort of a yes/no. "When you picture putting a juicy freshly cut lemon in your mouth, does it water?" Yes. And then she had me lie down and get comfortable, and she led me into my subconscious through hypnosis.

The few times I've been hypnotized, including this one, I always wondered if it was working. Yes, it worked. She led me to a hallway: What did it look like? It is lined with doors. Are they all the same or different? Is it light or dark? My hallway had dark, polished wood floors and all sorts of different doors on the left and sort of gothic-looking windows lining the right side of the hallway. The ceiling was grained and frescoed. She asked me to choose a door. The door I stopped in front of was made of dark, heavy, smooth wood, and the handle was metal and sort of in the shape of a cross. I pushed it open upon her suggestion.

Where was I? Was it dark or light? Warm or cold? Look down: Am I wearing shoes? What is the ground like? Look around: Where are you? I am in a forest clearing at night. It is warm, and I am looking at a big, beautiful tree. I am wearing boots, and the ground is very green. Grassy or mossy or some combination. I am wearing some kind of armor. I think maybe I'm a man because I'm a soldier, but then I realize I am not a man, I am a young woman of about twenty years old. I have long, wavy, strawberry blonde hair. And then Cozmo asks me to visit profound moments during this lifetime. In the first I was little, maybe about five, and in a small, modest cottage. My mother was giving birth, and it was very scary because there was a lot of blood and a lot of screaming. I'm not sure if she and the baby survived. Cozmo asks how I feel to be leaving that scene. I feel happy to leave it because it is scary.

In the next scene, I am about fourteen years old, underneath a big, beautiful tree, maybe the same one I recalled earlier, with a boy my age I love. I know that this boy is the man in my life now. We are flirting and kissing a bit. We are skipping stones on a pond or lake. I feel happy. When Cozmo asks me to leave this scene, I feel sadness because I know I won't see him again in this lifetime.

And then I am in battle on top of a white horse. This isn't as clear, perhaps because war and hand-to-hand combat isn't clear. I'm pretty sure I am killing or have killed people with my sword. There is a lot of adrenaline; I am fighting for my life and a cause larger than my own life, something I believe in. It is some battle for truth and light and freedom from oppression. When I leave this scene, I feel relief because it was an intense scene.

The next moment Cozmo leads me to is my death in that lifetime. Very quickly, I see myself struck down on the battlefield. It's as if I am watching from above. I see my body on the ground in my armor and regalia. I am sprawled out on the grass, and I am dead. There are some other soldiers around me. Although it has been the scene of great fear in the chaos of battle, there is something peaceful about it.

Cozmo brings me into a white, warm light. Who is there? I see my children and other family members and loved ones from this lifetime, some who are alive and some who have already passed on. She calls in angels and guides. I am aware of Archangel Michael, who brandishes a sword and is a great protector. She asks for them to share any messages with me. I chuckle out loud when I hear, "This lifetime, your pen is your sword." The message is clear to me that although I had to resort to violence in that lifetime to share and promote truth, healing, and freedom, I do not in this lifetime. I forgive myself for those acts of violence I committed in that lifetime, and I also recognize that I will not be killed for speaking the truth and shining a light in this lifetime.

Cozmo then guides me to leave this lifetime. We go out the way we came in. She leads me up the same staircase I descended, and I approach the door and open it, entering the long hallway with the dark wood floor once again. Cozmo asks me to mark this door somehow if this is a lifetime I would like to revisit. And then she counts me out of my hypnotic state, and I am awake and alert to this lifetime and my three-dimensional surroundings again.

She encourages me not to speak too much but to write about the experience. Even if things don't make sense, they might in time; they are clues, and it is as if we are putting together a puzzle. Also, she says I should pay attention to dreams and symbols that appear to me over the next three to seven days. She explains that although these symbols are always here and present, we are usually not in as receptive a state to truly see them. Cozmo also credits writing as one of the practices that helped and continues to help her significantly in her own healing. Getting into a flow state, not judging, not trying to fix or sort out anything—just more of a stream-of-consciousness style of writing.

This past life regression experience with Cozmo allowed me another way to integrate pieces of memory and own that part of myself, while also allowing me to forgive myself and others in my history for having committed acts of aggression in the past. My friend Kito offered a profound interpretation: "So often in fairy tales, it is the man who rides in on the white horse to rescue the woman. I love that you rode in on your own white horse and rescued yourself." I love that, too. I began to see themes emerge in all of these different modalities, showing me strong aspects of myself such as the female knight and the protective gorilla, while also becoming aware of other aspects/times that I have been a healer, a "witch," and a warrior fighting for light and healing and getting killed for it so many times. And recognizing that in this lifetime, I am safe.

FOR YOU:

Cozmo offers one-on-one sessions via her website, nikicozmo.com, and she also has guided meditation-like rituals for such goals as "release," "forgiveness," and "self-love." Weiss has some guided meditations and regressions you can download for a nominal fee from his website, brianweiss.com.

Who is it right for? Wrong for?

Past life regression might be particularly helpful for people who have already done a lot of healing work yet feel like there is something under the surface they can't quite access or release. It can also be a tool for better understanding certain relationships in this lifetime. It might not be a good fit for anyone with a diagnosed mental illness.

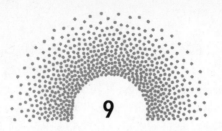

9

Integrating Trauma's Gifts

Every healing practice emphasizes the value of integration. In fact, much of the research on healing shows that healing can't take place until a traumatic experience is integrated. In order to heal, we must be whole and feel whole. Only we can make ourselves whole. There is no healer, lover, parent, child, friend, job, or accomplishment that can make us whole. Certainly supportive, loving, wise relationships and creativity can foster a fertile environment for us to identify, accept, and eventually love all aspects of our whole self. We are not whole if there is a part of us we have shut down, pushed aside, splintered off—a part resulting from trauma that perhaps is maladaptive, continuing behaviors that kept us safe during the trauma but are no longer useful and might now even be harmful. If we are avoiding certain places, people, or activities that trigger us about the trauma, it is a good indication we haven't yet integrated it.

The goal of healing, and I have found that my healing is ongoing, is getting to a place where we can remember and reflect on our traumatic history without it triggering a stress or fear response. It has simply become part of our history—an event in a series of events that has made us the people we are today, helped shape us, strengthened us, showed us parts of ourselves we didn't know prior to the trauma—an event or series of events without a label of "bad" or "good." I believe that is where the true healing lies, if we can somehow reach beyond the state of duality to accept, embrace, alchemize, and integrate it all because it just *is*.

I'm aware when I meditate, and was when I experienced ketamine therapy, of the question: Who is the "I" observing the "I" who is having a feeling, sensation, or reaction? Or even, who is that "I" of the past in that traumatic memory versus the "I" reflecting on it now? When I tap into this awareness, it allows me to recognize a larger, more connected "I" than the one I am often operating as—a wiser, more expansive, connected "I." Some spiritual teachers refer to this as my Higher Self or consciousness. Call it whatever you wish, but I make a practice to come from and with *that* Mary's perspective as much as possible. She makes much better choices; responds instead of reacts; doesn't experience as much judgment; and is calm, loving, and peaceful. And therefore the world she creates for herself is beautiful, abundant, joyful, and full of love.

Shortly after the mudslide, when I was in this state of connection with myself and with everything around me, I was astounded to witness my ability to manifest so specifically and quickly. I wasn't even aware at the time of what I was doing until after things I had wished for kept happening and appearing. This state of rawness, vulnerability, and purity in the aftermath of the mudslide was precarious and challenging, but it also felt like a magnificent door to connection with the divine had opened. It is always there and always open, yet we are often so distracted and disconnected from ourselves and our own divinity that we forget it's there and don't access it. I think my powerful ability to manifest while in this state was in part because of my heart and soul overriding my ego and intellect. I was so raw and so open, and the background noise of "life" had been blotted out as the true meaning of living demanded my attention. I would hope for things, and they would happen: Living in my dream house for a few weeks; then living around the corner from my sister in a house I was able to rent before I bought it, as I had wished. I began to be very conscious of my desires, my thoughts, and my language!

I began to investigate: How could I access this state regularly after I felt healed and no longer so raw? How can we stay in touch with the power of being broken open when we are no longer broken? How can we keep alive the resonance and compassion that often come in the aftermath of community trauma?

Here are some of my tools, strategies, and simple practices to keep in touch with the gifts following a trauma.

- Make choices about how you use language. Reframe your language about yourself and the role you played in the trauma. Practice referring to yourself as a "survivor" rather than a "victim."

- Eliminate the word "try" from your vocabulary; it's a word that sets you up to fail or not follow through.

- When you give your word to yourself, keep it. If you are not going to do something, don't say you are going to, for *you* above all else. If you break your word to yourself, you are giving yourself the message that it's not worth keeping, and you will be more apt to have others treat you this way, too.

- Practice positive self-talk. Your words and thoughts can reconfigure your brain and create your reality.

- Use the third person during self-talk; for example, "Mary can do this!" instead of "I can do this!" University of Michigan psychology professor Ethan Kross found that speaking in the third person bypasses the cognitive, effort-related part of the brain, having a direct positive effect by diminishing stress.

- Remember the law of attraction: In light of our ability to draw into our lives what we choose to focus on, imagine what you desire and not what you don't want to happen.

- Use rituals and visualizations for self-protection and alignment through focusing of energy, ideally when you are already relaxed, such as after meditating or exercising. To do this, sit or lie down with your eyes closed and visualize in as much detail as possible what you desire. If it's a beach vacation, smell the sea air, hear the seagulls, and feel the sand beneath your feet.

- Use essential oils, and smudge your space: Apply rose geranium essential oil to calm fear and burn palo santo or sage to clear and cleanse your home.

- Meditate, journal, and self-reflect.

- Stay wild: Spend time in nature playing, dancing, hiking, surfing, swimming, and expressing vibrancy and joy.

- Keep the right kind of company, with people who are encouraging, supportive, loving, uplifting, vulnerable, and growing.

- Limit exposure to news and media, including social media.

- Manage your time. Make and honor the time for your healing practices and rituals every day.

- Maintain emotional hygiene. Express your feelings, all of them, in a healthy way and environment. Be kind and honest with yourself and others.

- Intentionally create and maintain an inspired physical environment. Keep your space neat and tidy, make your bed, cut or buy flowers, open the doors and windows whenever possible to allow in fresh air, and display art that makes you feel good.

RELATIONSHIPS IN THE WAKE OF TRAUMA

Integrating our trauma personally is one facet. Our integration of it and how that factors into our relationships is another. Relationships with our family, friends, colleagues, and lovers make up the constellation of our lives. Author and spiritual teacher Mark Nepo puts it beautifully: "Life has been made just difficult enough that we need each other. The difficulty ensures the journey of love." How we give and receive love, or don't, how we learn and teach, how we define ourselves in relation to others all matter. The people we surround ourselves with correlates to how we feel. Take inventory of the seven people you spend the most amount of time with because they are a reflection of you. If you don't like what you feel, it's time to make some changes!

Our relationships can be areas in which we play out or heal unresolved and unintegrated trauma. Often, we choose partners who help us play out some unfinished pattern from childhood. Sometimes this can be healthy, and other times it's destructive. If we suffered abuse of any kind (physical or emotional) in our homes as children, we might unconsciously seek out an abusive partner in adulthood. Unless we work to identify and heal the pain of being abused by the very people meant to protect us, that becomes our set point of familiarity, and we feel secure in the insecurity. Or we might go the other direction. It's not uncommon for women who have been sexually assaulted to seek out partners who also carry unhealthy views of sex and perhaps patterns of sexual anorexia. With this direction they have successfully (albeit unconsciously) created a dynamic void of intimacy that might retrigger earlier trauma. When the trauma is healed, their desire and ability to connect intimately is healthily integrated, allowing for these aspects to once again blossom.

This leads us to the inevitable, rather cliche truth: Sometimes we grow in a different direction than our partner does. Often when we do our healing work, we have epiphanies for our highest and best good and for the highest and best good in every part of our lives. These revelations can also shine a light on our current relationship and the ways in which it has helped us stay in an unhealthy pattern, probably quite unconsciously. If the pattern can't shift, and if both people do not awaken to a similar consciousness at the same time, the relationship has to end. Although it might appear like a failure when a relationship ends and causes sadness, if done with grace, moving on from a relationship that has taught you all it can in its current iteration is the best path forward for all concerned. Nepo shares a metaphor of a big boulder being dropped into a body of water; if it is dropped to one side of the couple, it can propel you in the same direction. Sometimes it gets dropped between you, and through sheer physics, you are thrown in different directions. You can't force anyone to see and grow; everyone does that in their own time.

I remember reading about this concept and feeling fearful over what it would mean for my marriage. Ultimately, though, for me, when I had woken up to how differently I had processed the mudslide trauma and what that meant for how I wished to love, be loved, live, appreciate, and serve in the world with the time I had left, an amicable separation and divorce from my partner of twenty years was the only path forward that felt true. Although it was not easy, it was also freeing to be true to what I knew to be best for us both and our children. We had played the parts we were meant to play with each other in that role, and now it was time to shift roles. Author and spiritual teacher Shakti Gawain helped me process my initial guilt and sadness over the end of my marriage:

> When you've learned a great deal by being with someone, the energy between you may eventually diminish to the point where you no longer need to interact on a personality level as much, or at all. We don't understand this, so we feel guilty, disappointed, and hurt when our relationships change form. . . . I have found

that changes in relationships can be less painful, and at times even beautiful, when we can communicate honestly and trust ourselves in the process.[1]

Even when individuals experience exactly the same trauma, they will process and recover from it differently. Going through trauma and its aftermath can create dramatic changes in personalities and worldviews. This can be confusing, polarizing, and isolating, especially when people who deeply care about each other fail to see eye-to-eye about what is happening and what needs to happen. How do you get clear on and communicate how you need to feel supported by those closest to you following a trauma?

Nepo's experience with certain friends was that they were so uncomfortable about his grief that they were not able to go there. It wasn't the friends' not wanting to go there that drove apart those friendships, but it was their inability to admit that they didn't know how to and were afraid to. He explains, "If they could have said, 'Your grief scares me. I don't know what to do,' then we could have gone there together."

For me, the trauma of the mudslide initially thrust me and my then husband closer together as we worked through the beginning stages of shock, grief, gratitude, and putting our life "back together." After the logistics were more in place, and I went deeper into my healing and research, the issues in our marriage became more apparent and impossible to ignore. The ways in which we had approached our healing had created a chasm too wide to close. The boulder had been dropped between us, and we were propelled in different directions. Again, I want to reiterate that this is not to be feared. Liberating yourself from an unsatisfying at best, abusive and controlling at worst relationship can be an incredible gift. In fact, it is another "heavenly pivot" moment when something hard or traumatic pivots us toward heaven. Heaven in this case might be thought of as greater love, joy, peace, support, creativity, and freedom.

For so many of us, it can be hard to know how to be with someone who has just experienced a trauma. Do we say anything? Or will that make it worse? It can be uncomfortable because on some level, those around us are imagining how they would feel if your trauma happened to them. This can be scary or retriggering for someone who has experienced even another form of trauma; the impermanence and fragility of life has once again reared its head. No matter how in control we think we are, or we strive to be, ultimately, we are not in control. And by the way, yes, it is always best to acknowledge someone's trauma, even if all you say is, "I'm thinking of you, and I don't know what to say."

Before the mudslide I was someone who really resisted asking for help because I didn't want to impose on anyone or thought I could and should just do it all myself. After the mudslide, when we had lost all of our belongings, including wallets, phones, clothing, computers, cars, and home, it was impossible not to need and receive help. So many friends, family members, and strangers were incredibly generous, thoughtful, and helpful. In receiving support, love, and help, I felt as if my capacity to love actually grew. As so many spiritual teachers espouse, the other half of truly giving love is in receiving the love of others. We can't just be giving all the time and not receiving; otherwise, we're missing the point. Not only do we feel good when we receive love but also we allow the giver to enjoy and delight in the giving.

One of the greatest gifts in surviving trauma for me was the hyperfocus I found and the ability to appreciate getting another chance at life. In recognizing this, I understand how precious my time and energy is. It is important to appreciate and reconnect with primary relationships, get crystal clear about who my "real people" are, and clear away falsely close relationships, which became easy to identify after the mudslide.

As we expand and grow, we might outgrow old relationships that aren't as interesting, supportive, or collaborative anymore; let them fall away, and don't waste time or energy feeling guilty about it. "Another experience often reported by trauma survivors is a need to talk about the traumatic events, which sets into motion tests of interpersonal relationships—some pass, others fail. They also may find themselves becoming more comfortable with intimacy and having a greater sense of compassion for others who experience life difficulties."[2]

Allow your awakened self to attract like-minded, like-hearted lovers, friends, and colleagues who are on your new wavelength. Psychologist Edith Eger explains, "When you're in a vulnerable position with limited energy, it is especially crucial to choose how to spend your time."[3] And with whom! Shed or allow established relationships to transform. Create the most exciting, nurturing, supportive, expansive network for yourself as possible.

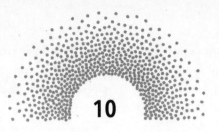

10

Radiant You

Now it is time to step into the rest of your life as the evolved, expanded, initiated, and extraordinary being you are! Remember your call to action and commitment to staying on the healing path that brought you to this book, which is always here to support you. Because each of us is unique, there is not an all-encompassing "prescription" for healing, so adapt and adopt from what is offered here. Most importantly, whatever practice you devise that works for you, make time for it. Honor yourself and your healing by making the time. As with going to the gym for your physical body, maintaining emotional and spiritual health also requires attention, time, focus, and commitment. Especially on the days and during the times in your life when everything feels great, stay with your practice. It will help make the dips less frequent and gentler. Again, create a practice and tailor a program that works for you.

As an offer of inspiration, I share mine as a springboard for you here and in greater detail at the end of this chapter. It begins with my internal dialogue upon waking; application of essential oils followed by a short qigong sequence; a morning meeting with myself and the Divine; physical exercise and movement; meditation; and a gratitude practice before bed, all to maintain healing and optimal health on the physical, emotional, and spiritual levels. These practices are here to ground and support you as you blaze your path forward into your glorious future.

Being aware of fear responses from ourselves and others is a good way to simply notice them and recognize them for what they are so as not to get tripped up by them. These negative thoughts and patterns are reactive, and they are just fear, so as hard as it may be, recognize them as that and move on. Two of the biggest ones I personally grapple with and hear the most follow.

THE OPINIONS OF OTHERS

"You're just lucky." I've heard this from friends and strangers alike about myself and others who have thrived in the wake of healing. Everything just seems to work out for you; you're so lucky. Enduring suffering, pain, misfortune, and trauma is part of being alive. As Edith Eger, a leading therapist on resilience training and posttraumatic stress disorder (PTSD) who survived Auschwitz, shares, "We are all likely to be victimized in some way in the course of our lives. At some point we will suffer some kind of affliction or calamity or abuse, caused by circumstances or people or institutions over which we have little or no control. This is life." She emphasizes that what we do have is the choice about how we respond to it. That puts us in the present moment of choosing our path forward.

How do you want to feel in the present? In the future? The "luck" comes in the choice to reframe the trauma and the healing practices around making the choice to thrive. Luck is work. It takes practice and effort to stay in a positive and heart-centered state of being. Going to the gym or an exercise class to work on our physical bodies is such an acceptable method of release and discipline; it is encouraging that spiritual practices are becoming more mainstream. So you see, it is not just luck—it is choice, focus, discipline, and practice.

I DON'T HAVE TIME

I get it! I have often thought this because I have two small children needing my attention; work to do; friendships; and constant cleaning, cooking, or tending to someone or something. I have had the thought of how easy it would be to have a greater spiritual practice if you live alone or have older children. And then in that moment, I had another epiphany: "This *is* the spiritual practice." Staying calm and grounded and loving in the face of life and unpredictability—*that's* the practice, and again why it is so important to do on a regular basis.

DAILY PRACTICE

As a way of integrating all of the facets of the modalities that have resonated and been most effective for me, I have a daily practice that I follow diligently to keep me in a balanced and harmonious state. I find it's important to be consistent. Do it on the days and during periods of life when things are going well and life feels joyful and easy, so that the inevitable lows are not as low, nor do they last as long. It's like going to the gym, staying fit and healthy—keep at it.

Wake up!

When I wake up, I take several deep breaths and think a version of, "This is going to be an incredible day. How can I express and feel more love today?" After washing my face and getting dressed, I practice qigong for twelve minutes to balance my nervous system and ground my energy. Hopefully, I've awoken before my children and can do it then, but otherwise, I'm doing it in the kitchen while they eat breakfast.

Morning Meeting

A "morning meeting" is a confluence of several teachings and books I have absorbed over the years. May McCarthy and *The Path to Wealth* was a great inspiration and jumping-off point that has morphed into practicing gratitude and setting my energy and intentions for the day. After dropping the kids off at school or while they watch cartoons on the weekend, I take about twenty to thirty minutes to meet with myself and God. I start by reading a short passage from an inspirational book. Two books I love are *The Collected Works of Florence Scovel Shinn* and *Ask and It Is Given* by Esther and Jerry Hicks. These two are great because they remind us how and why to focus our minds and thoughts on the positive. Where our energy and attention go, our energy flows. Basically, what we think, we create in our reality. If you are checking out right now and writing this off as woo woo, let's remember that this is quantum physics. Science. As Joe Dispenza explains in *Becoming Supernatural*, our attention is what creates something known as a "quantum event" or "collapsing the wave function." Essentially, physical matter (made of electrons) can't exist until we observe it, give it our attention. The moment we no longer put our attention on it, it turns back into energy, which scientists call a wave.[1]

After reading for a few minutes and generating or amplifying a good feeling, I open a journal (I have ones exclusively devoted to my morning meetings) and begin to write. For you, this could be a letter from your heart and soul to some higher power than yourself—God, if that feels right to you, or the Universe, the Divine, your Higher Self, Source, your Divine Team of Light—whatever works for you. Write the letter offering thanks for manifested reality you desire *already having happened.* For example, if you desire a beautiful new home, you would write, "Thank you for my gorgeous new home, which is mine by divine right." If there is a specific property you have in mind, include that, and always be sure to end with, "or something better." I am always sure to give thanks and write my desires with the caveat "with ease and grace" and/or "for the highest and best good of all concerned." Before the mudslide, I was asking for greater abundance often. I didn't ask for it with ease and grace. I did wind up with money from the insurance company, but that was not an easy or gracious process through which to receive abundance!

I also recommend not asking for things like patience. As Oprah Winfrey shared on one of her fantastic *Super Soul* podcasts, the year she asked for patience, she was given opportunity after opportunity to have to be patient. So, be careful how you write your letter. If there is something you desire that you don't yet have, write as if you already have it and are giving thanks. The idea here is to focus and calibrate your energy to the feeling of having it so that you can be a vibrational match for what you desire. What so many of us often do instead is focus on and feel the lack of what we desire. When we hold ourselves in the vibration of lack, we are not a match for having, so what we desire does not come to us! In the letter, start with true things and go from there. Here is an example of one of my morning letters:

> Dear God and my Divine Team of Light, Me,
> Thank you for a sound and restorative sleep. Thank you for this sunny morning, for birds chirping, for spring. Thank you for this beautiful room and house that feels like a cozy hug and is also spacious and inspiring. Thank you for my sweet, kind, well-behaved children and for my generous, thoughtful partner and our passionate and loving connection. Thank you for my vibrant, robust health and that of my family and community. I am grateful for the abundance in my life and having everything I need and desire with ease and grace. Thank you for my deal with XX closing on time for X amount of money or more for the highest and best of all concerned. Thank you for a record high

month of sales for the delight and happiness of all concerned, with ease and grace. I am grateful for exciting, fun, and expansive opportunities that are lucrative and help uplift others, myself included, with ease and grace. Thank you for gentle lessons. I am wealthy beyond my wildest dreams with over X amount of money in the bank to spend, invest, and grow, and shower upon those you and I see fit. Thank you for my divinely planned, protected, and financed travel to Europe and the Caribbean that is purely fun and joyful. For all of this and more and magic, I thank you and now I release these words to the law, truth, and power of the universe and it is done. Amen, and I love you!

After writing the letter, read it aloud. You have just set the tone and the energy for your day! In designing your day, revisit and review, add details, and practice staying with the emotions of gratitude and expectancy. For example, if one of your dreams is to go to a tropical island for a beach vacation, throughout the day see yourself on a white sand beach, the warm sun on your body, swimming in the turquoise waters. Buy a new bathing suit. Start noticing how you get feedback and encouragement as the trip comes together. Allow for that.

Having this practice in the morning really sets me up for being a happier, calmer, more productive version of myself throughout the day. Afterward, diving back into the role of mother, partner, friend, and business owner becomes easier and downright joyful most days. And other days, I'm grateful to have given myself a larger bandwidth! Depending on what is on the calendar that day, when I find time to complete my other practices varies.

Exercise

Most days I find time to move my body, which in turn often helps move stagnant emotion and thoughts out. Whether it's going to a favorite yoga class, hiking, going on a walk, taking a strength training class, or doing an online dance class, even if it's just for twenty minutes, I perceive a noticeable shift in my energy and mood and a healthier body. You can also turn on music and dance or shake your body while making dinner!

Qigong

Qigong is an ancient Chinese practice I describe in chapter 6. Refer to chapter 6 for more information and/or to incorporate the movements outlined there.

Meditate

Usually in the afternoon, I do a twenty-minute or longer meditation. I have practiced transcendental meditation off and on for years, and I also love Dispenza's meditations.

Before Bed

I do another quick qigong sequence before climbing into bed. This helps dispel any disharmonious energies from the day. After I'm in bed, I close the day by thanking God/the Universe/my Higher Power/Source (again, whatever works) out loud for various aspects of my day. I then say two forgiveness prayers—one asking to forgive anyone from my past whether I remember them or not, and the second forgiving anyone in the present, myself included. If there's anything more that needs to be communicated or help requested, I will do a final prayer.

I know it sounds like a lot, but after you start, it becomes easier and easier, and most days I truly look forward to it all because it feels good. I'm also actively creating my reality and a life that I love. I wish this for you, too! It might sound like a lot, so perhaps start by incorporating one new practice at a time that you can commit to, ideally for thirty days, and you can add more from there. The point is not to be overwhelmed but to find and tailor a daily practice that works for you!

RISING

Like a lotus blossoming out of the mud and a phoenix rising from the ashes, in history, art, and literature the preciousness, beauty, creativity, and wonder that comes from hard and messy things have been captured and celebrated. You are a miracle to be captured and celebrated. You made it through whatever trauma tested you. You are on the other side of it. You made it. You are safe, you are whole, and you are more dynamic, resilient, and brilliant than you were before. You most certainly didn't survive those experiences to go back to life as usual. You survived your trauma to soar, to follow your dreams, to recognize and embrace the fact that life is wild and precious and fleeting, so go on, live yours, and live it with as much joy and love as possible. Dawn has broken. The new day, your new life, is before you.

Acknowledgments

I want to thank all of the first responders who came to the physical, emotional, and spiritual aid of all of those affected in the Montecito mudslide of January 2018. I also want to acknowledge the families who lost loved ones that day.

Orion Womack, thank you for rescuing me that chilly morning. India Orion bears your name, and we are forever grateful for your bravery, determination, brilliance, and kindness. I want to thank and acknowledge my family and friends who rallied around me and my family, housing us, clothing us, feeding us, and seeing to our emotional well-being in the aftermath. Cousin Andrew, Ivana, Brooks, Anja, and Shane, thank you for taking us in. Kito Cetrulo and Analise Maggio, thank you for outfitting us and seeing to our basic needs and delights. Bright Start preschool, thank you for taking Ever for extra days and for the community providing supplies for Ever. The Tuttles, thank you for housing us in the most glorious beach house. Ellen DeGeneres, thank you for the toys, clothes, baby gear, and friendship at the beach and beyond. The Princeton girls and Fishers Island community, thank you for all of the love, support, clothing, books, gear, and toys. Amanda Lee, thank you for relentlessly finding us home after home. Jennifer Tucker, thank you for love and support. The Miraval Magic crew, thank you for all of the love, manifesting, and magic. Katie Ford, thank you for your generous support and cozy cashmere. Frida Arth, thank you for your sage and funny advice and support. Rita Chan Donahoe, thank you for your friendship and help reconciling one home and creating a new one. Morgan Mainz, thank you for the beam that saved our lives and your support creating a new home. Savanna Bomer, thank you for stability, balance, love, and support. Samantha Wennerstrom, thank you for ensuring I was a chic refugee in Doen. Elise Loehnen and goop, thank you for necessities and little luxuries. Michelle Wenke, thank you for Monrow T-shirts and luxe sweatsuits for our whole family. Angela Scott, thank you for my Office of Angela Scott boots and flats. Jennifer Freed, thank you for providing me emotional and psychological relief through EMDR and astrology sessions and for your enduring friendship. Thank you also for believing in me and this book and introducing me to my fabulous agent, Coleen O'Shea. Thank you, Coleen, for tirelessly working with me and championing the work. Thank you to my wonderful editor, Diana Ventigmilia, a soul sister on this journey. Thanks to everyone at Sounds True for your support and guidance. Thank you to Melissa Lowenstein for your strategy, focus, and discipline. Thank you to Jenny Kramer, a brilliant writer herself, who helped me shape and refine myself and my work. And for our writers' group!

To all of the incredible agents of change and healing I had the privilege of working with in my healing, thank you! Kim Vincent, I couldn't have made it through without you. Jeff Becker, you opened my consciousness and heart to another dimension for profound healing. Joe Dispenza, your meditations caused the chaos that led to triumphant evolution. Thank you for your brilliance. Minka, Naada, Gianna, from before, during, and after, thank you for your healing gifts and your friendships. Paul Fraser, thank you for clearing and helping me claim my whole heart and a healthy mind, body, and spirit.

To my parents, Susan and John, thank you for your support, benevolence, enthusiasm, and love. To my sister, Lucy, thank you for being the longest love relationship of my life, and the best business partner and best friend I could ask for. To Napper Tandy, thank you for being a wonderful coparent to our inspiring, resilient, and soulful children, Ever and India. Ever and India, thank you for choosing me as your mom and teaching me about love, kindness, and presence every day.

Resources

There are many foods and supplements I like to keep on hand to support my health and feeling good in my body and spirit. Below are some items I always keep on hand.

STOCK YOUR KITCHEN

Walnuts—support the brain and kidneys

Parsley—boil and drink the broth to prevent a urinary tract infection

Cilantro—helps rid body of heavy metal buildup; lowers anxiety

Arugula—flushes the liver

Pears—stewed pears and their broth are excellent for any sort of cough or bronchial imbalance

Strawberries—excellent source of vitamin C; one strawberry has one hundred times the vitamin C of an orange

Mint tea—helps to drain unhelpful energy from the heart

Eggs—loaded with protein and B vitamins, and choline, which is great for the brain

Lemons and limes—I like to add them to my water because they help your body absorb more water

Coconut water—full of natural electrolytes

STOCK YOUR MEDICINE CABINET

Magnesium teas or creams—help promote relaxation and sleep

CBD bath bombs—for sleep and relaxation

Thieves essential oil— (from Young Living) to ward off all sorts of illness

Epsom salts—for relaxation and release of stagnant energy

Magnolia oil—for lightening the fear associated with trauma

Rose oil—for opening the heart; also excellent for the face

Beta-blockers—for mitigating fear

Coconut oil—for moisturizing; also a lubricant

Notes

INTRODUCTION

1. US Department of Veteran Affairs, ptsd.va.gov/understand/common /common_adults.asp.

PART 1: TRANSFORMATION

1. Jeffrey Kluger, "Domestic Violence Is a Pandemic Within the COVID-19 Pandemic," *Time*, February 3, 2021, time.com/5928539 /domestic-violence-covid-19/.

CHAPTER TWO: THE MIND, HEART, AND BODY IN TRAUMA

1. Michael B. First, "Psychiatry's List of Disorders Needs Real-Time Updates," *Stat*, December 2016, statnews.com/2016/12/12/psychiatry -dsm-update/.
2. Ali A. El-Solh, "Management of Nightmares in Patients with PTSD: Current Perspectives," *Nature and Science of Sleep* 2018, no. 10 (November 26, 2018): 409–420, ncbi.nlm.nih.gov/pmc/articles /PMC6263296/.
3. Richard J. Ross, "The Changing REM Sleep Signature of Posttraumatic Stress Disorder," National Library of Medicine, August 1, 2014, pubmed.ncbi.nlm.nih.gov/25083007/.
4. El-Solh, "Management of Nightmares in Patients with PTSD."
5. Edith Eger, *The Gift* (New York: Scribner, 2020), 178.
6. Rebecca Solnit, *A Paradise Built in Hell* (New York: Penguin Books, 2009), 55.
7. Solnit, *A Paradise Built in Hell*, 70.

CHAPTER THREE: THE REFRAME, AND WHY NOW?

1. S. Cadell, C. Regehr, and D. Hemsworth, "Factors Contributing to Posttraumatic Growth: A Proposed Structural Equation Mode," *American Journal of Orthopsychiatry* 73, no. 3 (2003): 279–287.

2. L. G. Calhoun and R. G. Tedeschi, "Posttraumatic Growth: A New Perspective on Psychotraumatology," *Psychiatric Times* 21, no. 4 (2004).

3. M. Rutter, "Resilience as a Dynamic Concept," *Development and Psychopathology* 24, no. 2 (2012): 335–344, pubmed.ncbi.nlm.nih .gov/22559117/.

4. Rutter, "Resilience as a Dynamic Concept."

5. E. L. Quarantelli, "An Assessment of Conflicting Views on Mental Health: The Consequences of Traumatic Events," in *Trauma and Its Wake: The Study and Treatment of Post-Traumatic Stress Disorder*, vol. 1b, ed. C. R. Figley (New York: Brunner-Mazel, 1985), 173–218.

6. Faith G. Harper, *Unf*ck Your Brain* (Portland, OR: Microcosm, 2017), 37.

7. R. G. Tedeschi and L. G. Calhoun, "Posttraumatic Growth: Conceptual Foundations and Empirical Evidence," *Psychological Inquiry* 15, no. 1 (2004): 1–18, doi.org/10.1207/s15327965pli1501_01.

8. Edith Eger, *Embrace the Possible* (New York: Scribner, 2017), 7.

9. Srini Pillay, "911: Can We Do More Than Remember?" *Psychology Today*, September 11, 2010, psychologytoday.com/us/blog/debunking -myths-the-mind/201009/911-can-we-do-more-remember.

10. "Richard C. Schwartz, Ph.D.—The Founder of Internal Family Systems," IFS Institute, ifs-institute.com/about-us/richard-c-schwartz-phd.

11. T. X. Fujisawa, M. Jung, M. Kojima, D. N. Saito, H. Kosaka, and A. Tomoda, "Neural Basis of Psychological Growth Following Adverse Experiences: A Resting-State Functional MRI Study," *PLoS ONE* 10, no. 8 (August 20, 2015), ncbi.nlm.nih.gov/pmc/articles /PMC4546237/.

12. Kathy Eldon, *In the Heart of Life* (New York: HarperCollins, 2013), 313.

13. Eldon, *In the Heart of Life*, 344.

CHAPTER FOUR: MOVE IT!

1. TRE for All, traumaprevention.com.

2. B. Holzel, J. Carmody, M. Vangel, C. Congleton, S. M. Yerramsetti, T. Gard, and S. W. Lazar, "Mindfulness Practice Leads to Increases in Regional Brain Gray Matter Density," *Psychiatry Research* 191, no. 1

(January 30, 2011): 36–43, ncbi.nlm.nih.gov/pmc/articles /PMC3004979/.

CHAPTER FIVE: NATURE!

1. Elizabeth A. Krusemark, Lucas R. Novak, Darren R. Gitelman, and Wen Li, "When the Sense of Smell Meets Emotion: Anxiety-State-Dependent Olfactory Processing and Neural Circuitry Adaptation," *Journal of Neuroscience* 33, no. 39 (2013): 15324–15332.

2. Jeremy Appleton, "Lavender Oil for Anxiety and Depression," *Natural Medicine Journal* 4, no. 2 (February 2012).

4. Kerry Grens, "Regularly Whiffing Essential Oils Can Retrain Lost Sense of Smell," *Scientist*, November 2016.

5. *Natural/bio-identical progesterone* refers to a form of this hormone molecularly identical to the stuff made by the body. It is not the same thing as the progestins one finds in oral contraceptives or synthetic hormone replacement drugs, molecules that are constructed to occupy progesterone hormone receptors in the body but that actually bear little resemblance to the hormone made by the body.

CHAPTER SIX: CHINESE MEDICINE

1. Yi Zhuang, "History of Acupuncture Research," *International Review of Neurobiology* 111 (2013): 1–23.

2. "Acupuncture," Johns Hopkins Medicine, hopkinsmedicine.org/health /wellness-and-prevention/acupuncture.

3. Michael Hollifield, "Acupuncture for PTSD: A Randomized Controlled Pilot Trial," *Journal of Nervous and Mental Disease* 195, no. 6 (June 2007): 504–513.

4. E. C. Ritchie, "Integration of Alternative Therapies Shows Promise in PTSD Treatment," *Healio*, April 17, 2013, healio.com/news/psychiatry /20130417/sargent_10_3928_1081_597x_20130401_15_1110401.

5. Lauren Hubbard, "What to Know About Gua Sha, the Old-School Crystal Skin Tools Taking Over Instagram," *Fashionista*, July 25, 2018, fashionista.com/2018/07/gua-sha-facial-tool-benefits.

6. Laura Johannes, "The Intriguing Healthy Benefits of Qigong," Harvard Medical School, September 30, 2013; Yufang Lin, "What Are the Health Benefits of Qigong?" Cleveland Clinic, September 23, 2020.

CHAPTER SEVEN: LET'S GET CLINICAL

1. Bessel van der Kolk, *The Body Keeps the Score* (London: Penguin, 2014), 251.
2. Garrett Hassett, "The Effectiveness of EMDR," Boston University, August 11, 2018.
3. Rachel Nuwer, "A Psychedelic Drug Passes a Big Test for PTSD Treatment," *New York Times*, May 3, 2021, nytimes.com/2021/05/03 /health/mdma-approval.html.
4. R. Nardou, E. M. Lewis, R. Rothhaas, R. Xu, A. Yang, E. Boyden, and G. Dolen, "Oxytocin-Dependent Reopening of a Social Reward Learning Critical Period with MDMA," *Nature*, April 3, 2019, nature .com/articles/s41586-019-1075-9.
5. Edward Edinger, *Ego and Archetype* (Boston, MA: Shambhala, 1992), 109–110.
6. Edith Eger, *The Gift* (New York: Scribner, 2020), 79.
7. American Group Psychotherapy Association, agpa.org/home.

CHAPTER EIGHT: INTO THE GREAT WIDE OPEN!

1. Sameer S. Chopra, "Industry Funding of Clinical Trials: Benefit or Bias?" *Journal of the American Medical Association*, July 2, 2003.
2. James Nestor, *Breath* (London: Penguin, 2020), 160.
3. Nestor, *Breath,* 163.
4. Nestor, 212.
5. Gabby Bernstein, *Super Attractor* (New York: Hay House, 2019), 95.
6. Maria Cohut, "Transcendental Meditation Can Help Treat PTSD," *Medical News Today*, February 20, 2019.
7. Bernstein, *Super Attractor,* 121.
8. Philip M. Ullrich and Susan K. Lutgendorf, "Journaling About Stressful Events: Effects of Cognitive Processing and Emotional Expression," *Annals of Behavioral Medicine* 24, no. 3 (2002): 244–250.
9. Shaman Durek, *Spirit Hacking* (New York: St. Martin's, 2019), 169.
10. Jonathan Goldman, *Jonathan Goldman's Healing Sounds* (Boulder, CO: Sounds True), healingsounds.com/overview-sound-healing/.
11. Emma Young, "Lifting the Lid on the Unconscious," *New Scientist*, July 25, 2018.

CHAPTER NINE: INTEGRATING TRAUMA'S GIFTS

1. Shakti Gawain, *Living in the Light* (Springfield, VA: Nataraj, 2011), 133.
2. L. G. Calhoun and R. G. Tedeschi, "Posttraumatic Growth: A New Perspective on Psychotraumatology," *Psychiatric Times* 21, no. 4 (2004).
3. Edith Eger, *The Gift* (New York: Scribner, 2020), 24.

CHAPTER TEN: RADIANT YOU

1. Joe Dispenza, *Becoming Supernatural* (New York: Hay House, 2017), 64.

About the Author

Mary Firestone has been a student of healing and living life to the fullest her entire adult life. After earning her BA in English from Princeton University and an MA in clinical psychology from Pepperdine University, she founded Firestone Sisters in 2012 with her sister, Lucy. The sisters produce and curate their Wild Precious Life Retreats with the aim of providing healing and growth opportunities for women both nationally and internationally. The Montecito mudslide was an acute crisis that furthered Mary's lifelong curiosity and commitment to healing, sharing what works for her, and self-development. The retreats have been written about on Goop, *Travel + Leisure, Santa Barbara Magazine,* Forbes Travel Guide, Well+Good, and *Angeleno.* Mary and Lucy have contributed to *Travel + Leisure, Angeleno, Jetsetter,* Passported, and the *Louis Vuitton City Guides.* They also produce an essential oil–based perfume called The First. Mary lives with her family in Santa Barbara.

About Sounds True

Sounds True is a multimedia publisher whose mission is to inspire and support personal transformation and spiritual awakening. Founded in 1985 and located in Boulder, Colorado, we work with many of the leading spiritual teachers, thinkers, healers, and visionary artists of our time. We strive with every title to preserve the essential "living wisdom" of the author or artist. It is our goal to create products that not only provide information to a reader or listener but also embody the quality of a wisdom transmission.

For those seeking genuine transformation, Sounds True is your trusted partner. At SoundsTrue.com you will find a wealth of free resources to support your journey, including exclusive weekly audio interviews, free downloads, interactive learning tools, and other special savings on all our titles.

To learn more, please visit SoundsTrue.com/freegifts or call us toll-free at 800.333.9185.

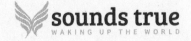